MW00510765

DANCING
Out
OF THE CLOSET

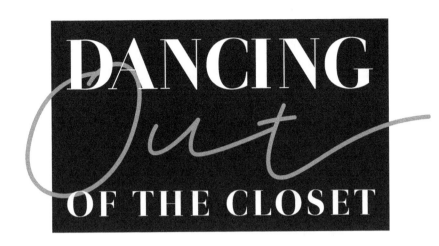

DANCING
Out
OF THE CLOSET

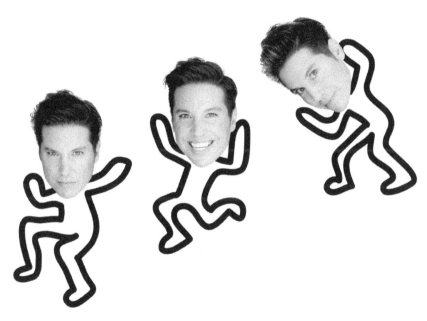

TOTALLY TRUE STORIES
BY
MATTHEW SHAFFER

BearManor Media
2019

Dancing Out of the Closet

© 2019 Matthew Shaffer

All rights reserved.

Published in the United States of America by:

BearManor Media
P. O. Box 71426
Albany, GA 31708

BearManorMedia.com

Printed in the United States.

Typesetting and layout by John Teehan

Front & Back Cover Author Head Shots: @russell.baer

ISBN—978-1-62933-455-4

Jeffrey, you will always be my little bug. Kellyn,
may you never feel compelled to hide.
I love you both unconditionally.

Contents

Author's Note

What do politicians, lawyers, and artists have in common? Actually, please don't answer that question. My self-esteem can't handle the plethora of insults that have certainly started swirling in your mind about people who exaggerate the truth to prove a point.

Much like a young child who recounts the events of a schoolyard tiff to the principal, leaving out details that might cause personal damage; artists tend to examine life through an emotional magnifying glass. Embellishing when it helps build drama, adding a punch line to a circumstance in order to lighten the tone, and perhaps withholding evidence when it might cause unnecessary destruction.

The events and stories I share in this book are based on my career in the entertainment industry and my journey of self-discovery. Some situations and names have been reinterpreted (as artists often do) in an effort to spare the ego of an unsuspecting person who happened to come in contact with me on my adventure. I offer my hard earned memories as inspiration and entertainment. If you feel that you've been slighted by my recollection, I encourage you to share your side of the story in your book.

Acknowledgements

People assume Hollywood types are all selfish, and they're correct. Occasionally, we find room to let someone else talk. I recognized very early in my career that, as fabulous as I knew I was, I perform better with a co-star. Jeff, thank you for setting me up to succeed in every adventure we embark on. You enrich every aspect of my personal and professional life. Thank you for being my creative editor, motivating me to dig deeper, and for sharing the stage.

In Hollywood *everyone* has an agent, manager, lawyer, and publicist. (Most of us have a guru and a "good" doctor, too, but that's not my point.) Michelle Zeitlin has spent the past 15 years pounding down doors and navigating my "crazy." Together, with Jeff, we have laughed, cried, pitched, failed, triumphed, and relentlessly pursued our purpose. I cannot imagine a career without you. Thank you for supporting me. Fighting for me. Talking me off (many) ledges, and never giving up on me. I used to think success would come for us and we'd be laughing our way to an acceptance speech. Now, I'm certain that success is found entirely in the company we keep and the adventures we share together. From my POV you remain: The World's Best Manager.

Jane Hamilton, thank you for coming on board and lending your insight, passion, and energy.

It's no secret that our loved ones have a remarkable talent for penetrating our boundaries despite their best effort to express love or concern. Which explains why I use the self-help section at Barnes & Noble as my own personal therapy retreat at least once a week. It's free and they serve Starbucks coffee—enabling both my addiction to caffeine and collecting inspirational quotes from people whose names I cannot pronounce. Still, I would be nothing without the unending love and support of my entire family. Thank you for tolerating me on my journey of self-discovery. I am aware that I made things challenging and still you remained supportive of my dreams. I apologize for thrusting you onto the page unwillingly, but my story wouldn't be the same without you. Specifically, to my Mom and Steve, Dad and Louise, Abby, Shiree, and Kellyn—I love you.

To my cousin, *Bryan*, I understand the magnitude and appreciate your bravery for allowing me to share our story. I'm so proud of you, and hope that our journey will ease the path for someone in a similar circumstance.

Christine Paynton, your love, generosity, and encouragement are endless. To my in-laws; I cherish each of you.

I'm always grateful to workshop my material, and the fierce artists in my writers' group inspired and motivated me whilst sifting through the rubble. Thank you: Julietta Corti, Anthony J. Marciona, Joseph A. LoBue, Joanne DiVito, Carolyn Dyer, and Tam Warner. You nourished me every step of the way.

Jacqueline C. Riggs, thank you for embracing my direction and allowing me to shine.

Mr. Osburg, the look on your face after my wretched audition at the 9th grade drama competition continues to humble me.

Nan and Gus Giordano, thank you for providing me with my entrance into the world of professional dance.

To *Daniel*, I'm sure you're unhappy about unknowingly becoming a major character in my "play," I hope wherever you are, you've found peace. Thank you for helping me out of the closet.

To *Kristen*, I'm sorry that I hurt you.

Ben and everyone at BearManor Media, thank you for this extraordinary opportunity and for all of the guidance, wisdom, and patience along the way.

Thank you to my editor, Aidan Cross, without whom readers would discover just how creative I am with my spelling and grammar. To my typesetter, John Teehan, for helping my words pop off the page with his dazzling layout.

Some people never judge a book by its cover. For the remaining 99% of us, I'm elated to know George Skinner. George, your artistic abilities are unbounded; thank you for nailing my book cover design!

Finally, to my village:

Jen Toby, Torri Oats, Sandy Coyte, Grace Wakefield, Bevin Allen, Brooke and Todd Cooper, Tracie Stanfield, Bruce Martin, Matthew and Mary Beth Lodes, Melissa and Marc Johnson, Maria Tucker, Christelle Nesbitt, Amy Claire, Logan Sparks, Ellen and Brian Dreyfuss, Jeffrey James Shoe, Janis Faye, Lisa and Terry Lindholm, Beckie King, Ari Warshawsky, Samuel Roberts, Sylvia Lane, Chris Clarkin, Lesley Wolff, Jennifer Oliver O'Connell, Michelle Loucadoux-Fraser, Valerie Smith, and Catherine Handy;

THANK YOU!

(VERY) Foreword

I know what you're thinking—a second book? This guy only sold two copies of his first book (thanks mom and dad), how narcissistic is he? Actually my literary debut, *So You Want To Be A Dancer*, launched as a #1 New Release in Performing Arts on Amazon and made a comical cameo on *The Tonight Show* with Jimmy Fallon. More importantly, it (momentarily) quenched my Kathy Griffin-like appetite to over share twenty years of juicy Hollywood drama and boost my social media presence from the "D-List" to a respectable C+… it's all about the followers.

Despite the undeniable fact that I have achieved a healthy dose of self-love (thank you yoga, Eckhart Tolle, and daytime talk shows), I am NOT: self-centered, egotistical or self-obsessed as the Google search definition of the word "narcissist" would label me. Fine. I'll concede to the truth that I'm a skosh vain. I blame the "everyone wins a trophy", "snap a selfie and post it on Instagram" generation of which I am a product. Otherwise I'm a totally normal guy in my late-thirties (OKAY) early-forties, trying to find my place in Hollywood.

Why? Similar to most actor–dancer–writer–producer–comedian–choreographers, I adore attention. Of course it's about "the art", but it's also about someone gloating over me in the art.

It was only after writing this book and reliving the embarrassing and brutal reality of my childhood; the Desperately-Seeking-Fame quest of my early adulthood; and the wild "pinch me so I'll know I'm not dreaming" adventures I've had alongside stars like Leonardo DiCaprio, Adam Levine, Amy Poehler, or Rebel Wilson; when I realized that my life-long thirst for notoriety was less about becoming famous and more about the validation that comes with it. Not from Hollywood power players handing out awards, the fans, or even my family—but from myself.

I've spent my life searching for my own approval; yearning to stop dressing up, stop covering up, stop pretending, hiding, deflecting, overachieving… just stop! It was time to take a long hard look at myself in the mirror and face reality: I am GAY. Why–even in the 21st century—is it so terrifying for us to confront the personal obstacles that make us unique or label us as different?

I didn't grow up in an utterly dysfunctional family. I was never abused, nor was I emotionally deprived. Actually, I was spoiled with attention, praise, laughter, love, and positive reinforcement—so really I have my family to blame for my grossly humiliating display of vanity.

Is it my fault that at age nine I forced my sister and cousins to endure writers' meetings to discuss their lack of using ME in every sketch that we were collaborating on for our pre-YouTube camcorder production of *We're Too Sexy?* (A fabulous rip off of *In Living Color*, which was an even more remarkable rip off of *Saturday Night Live*.)

NO. Again, I blame my parents. If they weren't so ready to accept my eagerness to be an entertainer—or maybe just get me out of their hair—I wouldn't be the talented, hilarious, adorable, charming celebrity (in my own head) that I am today.

Still, I can't help my relentless attraction to the world of "show". My addiction to telling funny stories in a group of people to get a laugh, share a thought provoking comment on Facebook to arouse social engagement, or dawn a dress like a Bravo-lebrity and act out a digital short* with my husband (we will get back to the use of the word husband later in the book) to post on YouTube; adding to our millions of views. Seriously, are you following me on Instagram, yet?

So here I am tackling another book. Hey, I still want the fame; I'm dying to get a good table at Craig's without a reservation. Although, even after orchestrating and navigating through an unrelenting amount of emails, conference calls, and pitch meetings between my manager, agent(s), publicist(s), publisher, partner, and the media I

---

*   A digital short is a fancy way to say sketch in the hopes that a network will fall madly in lust with the content and hand us the keys to the television kingdom.

sincerely doubt I'll be elevated to Ryan Reynolds status overnight—God I wish I had his abs.

Hidden in all of us you'll discover a metaphorical closet where we've hoarded our darkest secrets, most irrational fears, and unresolved traumas. The parent who can no longer hide the inevitable divorce from their children; the addict who fights to come to terms with their substance abuse; the teenager who struggles with depression or an eating disorder. It was in my pursuit of becoming a professional dancer where I found the conviction, confidence, and creative expression to face my demons and the grace to dance through them.

The stories you're about to read represent the dancer in all of us, searching for a stage to dream on whether you are a doctor, lawyer, teacher, or stay-at-home-Superhero juggling between the carpool club, soccer practice, ballet classes, and baking lopsided—but delicious—cupcakes for the PTA. No matter who you are, you've undoubtedly rehearsed your OSCAR® acceptance speech, imagined receiving a Noble Peace Prize, or fantasized about capturing Olympic Gold. Face it—we all hope to win the lottery, even if we don't buy the tickets.

Thank you for picking up this book. I'm aware that you're auditioning me right now. With any luck, I've made it past the first cut. If so, meet me in the first chapter where we will begin a journey of self-acceptance. Together we'll save thousands of dollars on therapy. Oh, and congratulations! It's rare for people to read a book about a non-Kardashian, unless the author is a former President or a female comic-turned-Hollywood-It-Girl. Which is cool, so long as I'm able to get a third book deal out of this. Here we go!

Waiting

The indignation, which accompanies my abandonment *issues* can be traced all the way back to a very early childhood memory. Barely out of diapers, I was already functioning like a true professional. I preferred a legal pad to Lego's, which manifested into a bizarre fascination with paper products. By the time I was five years old the smell of a lead pencil scratching against a spiral bound notebook and the urge to be organized, seduced me into taking one of my grandma's used day-planners.

Back when a telephone hung from a wall and a calendar sat on a desktop—which was actually made of wood—the heft of the pages in my hands, the visually stunning grids, and colorful tabs were much more agreeable with my personality than the plastic toys my peers were distracted with. It was in this primitive form of record keeping that I implemented a system of bold crayon colors to cover the already marked up book in order to keep track of my daily goals and activities, which included decorating the store-front window at my grandparents' liquor store (we'll discuss this later), color coordinating my corduroy jeans, and taking baths. I liked to be clean.

My parents were still in training pants when they had me; it was kind of like we were growing up together. My repurposed organizer was just one way that I could contribute to our household while maintaining a sense of control. My sister, who was still in diapers at the time, was somewhat of a renegade—fearless with an endless appetite for danger, adventure, and making my life hell.

I was completely caught off guard one Friday afternoon, when a routine visit to my grandparents' house turned out to be a strategically coordinated drop-and-dash date night for my mom and dad. How could this be? I may have been pintsized, but I knew that our overnight bags took some time to prep. Why wasn't I consulted before this decision was made? Why wasn't this labeled in red crayon on my calendar? And most importantly, dad, why are you wearing those cowboy boots with slacks?

After I delivered a twenty-five minute argument clearly articulating my concerns while highlighting incentives to include me on their evening of dinner, drinks, and dancing, the dictator (my dad) ordered me to a fifteen-minute time out on grandma's lap.

Naturally, I was unwilling to give up my fight so easily. I should have been a trial lawyer but instead I decided upon an acting career for one primary reason: as an actor, you can lie without swearing on the Bible.

The minute my right butt cheek touched down on my grandma's lap, I had worked up my first tear. I tried to win my case the adult route—with facts and reason—and that didn't get the job done. Now, I was going to have to act my age and deliver a full-blown outburst.

Some kids throw tantrums; but please trust me when I say that I do not do anything small. I pride myself on pure, unashamed emotional outbursts, which include: flailing around on the floor while kicking and screaming, pounding my head into walls, pulling my hair out, covering my mouth and depriving myself of oxygen, and my personal favorite – scratching my fingernails down the side of my face. The scene was similar to an event you might expect from a Kardashian if you suspended their Instagram account.

My compelling scene was so exquisitely staged that I'm positive it would have garnered my first Academy Award nomination. Sadly, I did not prevail. In my snot-covered fury, I missed the chance to give my mom and dad a hug goodbye.

During my signature fish flail, they snuck out the back door. In a melodramatic fashion, I pounded on the window that segregated me from my parents, who were near their car. Finally, my mom caved, turned back to face me, and shouted, "We'll be back to pick you up tonight, I promise."

I got her! Certain that the overnight bag they'd packed with care was going unused—I called back, "So we have a deal then? You promise, right?"

"I promise." She confirmed, again. Score one for me. I struck an agreement with my mom.

I watched their car drive off into the distance from the safety and comfort of my grandma's arms. I acknowledged that *this* was really happening, so I might as well make the most of my time with grandma and grandpa.

Grandma was a short, energetic, Italian Catholic with fine, snow-white skin, animated doe-eyes, a naturally thin physique, and an impeccably teased hairdo, which stayed perfectly coiffed when she slept thanks to her silk pillowcase. Her Faith was strong, but never conflicted with her wit, intelligence, business acumen, or feminist spirit.

Grandpa was James Dean good looking. He stood straight, but not ridged with a lean athletic frame, which gave the illusion that he was much taller than he was. Confident, wise, and perceptive, he knew exactly when to use his charismatic charm but contained his thoughts so that when he spoke, you listened.

My grandparents spent the evening spoiling us rotten. Gram was intuitive of my creative inclination and sought to rouse my imagination with craft projects. While my grandpa bounced my sister on his knee like she was riding in the Kentucky Derby, Gram and I spent two hours working on a project. Cutting construction paper, gluing glitter onto stars, and designing a sparkling display for the 4 x 6 window that faced Main Street where Shaffer's Still was located. Thanks to the encouragement of my Gram, I believed that I was conceptualizing the installation for a Bergdorf Goodman's holiday window display rather than for the family liquor store.

Following a delicious dinner (I can still smell the mouthwatering aroma of my grandma's spaghetti and meatballs) we were offered an endless buffet of cakes, muffins, candy, cookies, and soda.

My grandpa captivated us with a magic show, which included his classic finger split, an illusion that convinced us that his thumb had been detached from his hand. It was his grand finale—when he removed his teeth from his mouth—that left us in shock and awe for hours. It was brilliant.

Afterward, my grandma had to explain that children who eat too much candy growing up are forced to go to the dentist to have their real teeth replaced with a set of false teeth. This revelation only encouraged me to eat more of the sugary treats throughout the evening.

Following *Wheel of Fortune, Jeopardy,* and *Murder She Wrote,* my grandma read us a story in the hopes that we would get sleepy. She and my grandpa always laid out blankets on the floor of their bedroom, with comfy pillows next to their bed. While I loved the smell of the blankets and the security of knowing that I would be sleeping in a safe spot, I objected to falling asleep without holding my parents to their promise.

My grandma spent the entire evening holding me in her arms, singing to me in the rocking chair that sat next to their bed. I attempted to distract her and offset sleep by making up stories and reenacting monologues that I had heard during *Murder She Wrote.* I resisted sleep for what felt like hours, but was probably more like forty-five minutes. I woke up the following morning to the smell of candied coffee, buttery eggs, and fresh homemade bread; my grandma was waiting for me in the kitchen. I felt abandoned by my parents, and worse still, they'd lied to me!

Keen on my ultra sensitive emotional disposition and eager to refocus my attention on harnessing creative outlets rather than imploding, my grandma suggested we take a trip to the public library. We pulled up to the beautiful old municipal building with the large cement stairway leading up to the main entrance and I walked through hand-in-hand with my grandma. Immediately the bouquet of perfumed, slightly musty books hit me. Mountainous rows of knowledge towered over me in every direction. A very eccentric and boisterous librarian—who happened to be a close friend of my grandma's—greeted me with a big kiss on the cheek and handed me a stack of books that she had preselected just for me.

I couldn't wait to return to grandma and grandpa's house to crack open the plastic covered children's books; the bindings had been Scotch taped from years of wear-and-tear so I knew they must be good.

I would act out the scenes as gram read the stories from *Alice In Wonderland, The Giving Tree,* and *The Wizard Of Oz.* Occasionally, my gram would pause to pull out a wooden spoon and a kitchen towel, which she fashioned as a cape and scepter. She added these props to layer my theatrical experience, deepen my imagination, and flare my fantasy.

My grandmother understood me entirely. Perhaps because of our Taurus birthdays, which fell just two days apart from one another, or because she was the most extraordinary, generous, insightful person I've ever met. She empowered my delicate personality and helped me escape my self-inflicted torment through laughter, love, and a lot of overly salty Italian meats, cheeses, and sugary cookies loaded with lard.

My parents returned to collect my sister and me around noon, but by then the damage had been done. Their innocent date night was the beginning of my thirty-year battle with trust, rage, abandonment, and addiction to finding comfort through food. It was also the moment my gram became my very best friend.

Four Eyes

Anyone can see the glitter bouncing off my brilliantly-maintained mane now that I've long departed the land of self-hate and accepted what was obvious to everyone else around me: I was meant to sparkle.*

Like so many of the coming out stories we gays share around the penis-shaped punch bowl at Liza Minnelli's house, my childhood was a delicate balancing act in the art of hiding from the truth, while belting out a show tune, and denying an attraction to Kirk Cameron (The *Growing Pains* years, not the Jesus crusade).

I grew up in a supportive middle-class Catholic home with very young parents who were raising themselves and their two children, while playing house. My mom, a beautiful, smart, witty woman with a love for shopping—was a delightful escape from my inner voice. My dad, a handsome, wise, hot-headed man with a passion for the outdoors and being right in every circumstance, was the perfect model for my attempt to fit in with the boys my age. Both of my parents were nurturing and loving above everything else, so I had no reason to loathe myself so much.

I knew I was not in love with the ingénue of fifth grade, Hazuki Akemi, but *she* was in love with Jeff Menrou, the tow-headed, surfer-jock with a bright smile; thus began my secret crush. I sat in the third row in Mrs. Trevor's fifth grade class—two rows behind the girl who would become my prime adolescent obsession.

---

* Please note that my line reading of "sparkle" is with a big gay lisp (not because I have one) but because I am gay and not afraid to use it when emphasizing a point for dramatic effect.

Every closeted gay boy eventually realizes that he needs a bestie beard with whom to socialize at lunch, jump rope, swing on the monkey bars, and get close to cute boys without raising suspicions. Who better than the smartest, most popular Asian beauty at Joseph Arnold Elementary School?

My plan was simple yet foolproof: Become friends with her (not-yet-out-in-fifth-grade-but-totally-obvious) gay best friend, Rob. They played tetherball together every day during our first recess and I would work my way into the rotation and rope Rob out.

Too bad my plan failed—it turns out I'm terrible at tetherball. Rob and Hazuki had no time to waste on my (then) lack of ball skills.

Fortunately, around the same time, the California School Board decided square dancing was a positive way to socialize young boys and girls about the mysteries of the opposite sex.

I found my way in—I was already incredibly passionate about dance—and I was all set to impress Hazuki (and subsequently, but also more importantly, Jeff) with my master moves.

Every Friday after lunch, both fifth grade classes would meet in our multi–purpose cafetorium. Here one could play basketball, rehearse for the school musical, eat lunch, endure a D.A.R.E. assembly, and learn the basic steps of American Square Dancing, all in one place.

After two classes, I was ready to take my act on the road. While everyone else was busy trying to breakdown a box step, I was allemande left-ing my way to the pros and soon into the arms of Hazuki, or so I hoped. Four weeks into square dancing lessons, I was still riding hay while the other boys twirled Hazuki around the room.

Okay, so I'm aware that I haven't confronted the obvious question here: If you had a crush on the cute blond surfer boy, why were you so consumed with Hazuki? The answer is simple. If I couldn't *have* Jeff, I didn't want Hazuki to get him either. I had to devise a stronger, more elaborate plan. Or, at least be close to the girl that did have him.

After talking to Sarah Colby, the class informant, I learned that Hazuki was only interested in dating boys who wore glasses; because she herself wore glasses and felt that it was an important requirement.

It was going to be a challenge to convince my parents to buy me prescription glasses in order to impress a girl from my class only to get cozy with Jeff Menrou. Certainly I couldn't come right out and ask my mom to take me to the optometrist, "Mom, there's a girl in my class who will only date boys that wear glasses. I really need this girl to like me. This would no doubt have an impact on my popularity—you want me to be popular, right?"

I opted for a more subtle and elaborate approach, which would require a significant amount of time, energy, and dedication. I was up for the challenge, because I knew it meant a solid social foundation for my transition to Callé Mayor Middle School.

Day One, I rose my hand during Mrs. Trevor's explanation of the three branches of government. From my third row seat near the back of the room, I could clearly make out: Judicial, Legislative, and Executive, but Hazuki needed a studious lover, and that's what she was going to get.

"Mrs. Trevor?"

"Yes, Matthew—what can I help you with?"

"I'm sorry, I'm just having a little trouble reading your writing—can you please tell me what the third word is?"

"Yes, it says Executive—which is what I was in mid-discussion about before you interrupted."

"Thank you."

The seed was planted. Over the course of the semester, I continued to feign difficulty making out words; I complained about habitual headaches; during our group reading circles I would pause dramatically, and squinted my eyes when I got to a word that was larger than four letters; in the middle of presenting a book report, I would stop and apply pressure to my temples; when a teacher was near, I never missed an opportunity to express difficulty identifying an object.

Finally, Mrs. Trevor took the bait, "Matthew, can you please come here for a moment?" *This is it!* I felt giddy inside as I made my way toward Mrs. Trevor's desk and passed Hazuki, who was quietly working on her essay with her darling Hello Kitty pencil box perfectly organized.

"You wanted to see me?"

"Matthew, I've noticed that you have been having a lot of trouble reading and focusing. I'm concerned that you might need some extra attention."

"Oh no, it's nothing like that Mrs. Trevor—I just can't see very well, and I've been getting really bad headaches."

"Have you mentioned this to your parents?"

"No, I don't want to bother them—my sister just got braces and I know they're worried about money." I felt bad about lying and terrible about throwing my parents under the bus like that—but my vision of the future just became clear; Hazuki wants a four-eyed surfer, that's what I'm giving her!

"Take this to the nurse's office and she will help you with this *situation*." Just like that, Mrs. Trevor had become a collaborator in my optical quest for the forbidden romance.

The nurse's office was a familiar place for me—I was a frequent client of the vinyl-padded bed covered in butcher paper. It was a safe place to escape the trials of recess bullies and pop quizzes in math class.

I bypassed the secretary, who sat behind the main office desk and proceeded directly to the "waiting room," which consisted of two school chairs that sat directly in front of the all-in-one nurse's station, complete with an eye-flushing kit, a bucket of EpiPens, and a jar of tongue depressors.

Side note: I would become very familiar with the eye-flushing kit my second year of middle school after an incident in Woodshop that involved liquid glue, a paint brush, and a substitute teacher; more on this story later.

The hospital curtain was drawn, which meant Nurse Nancy had a client—most likely Elana Edgmont. She frequented the nurse's office more than Lindsay Lohan relapsed into rehab. I'm positive the girl had a punch card.

I waited impatiently, tapping my foot on the green-and-white-checkered linoleum floor to alert the nurse that she had company. Unlike Elana's undoubtedly false "girl troubles", I had a serious *situation,* which was legitimized by Mrs. Trevor. After what felt like two hours, Nurse Nancy slung open the curtain and smiled when she saw my face, "Mr. Shaffer, to what do I owe the pleasure."

I handed her my note like a defense lawyer for the Trial of the Century. "As you can see from Mrs. Trevor's note, I'm having extreme difficulty focusing in class. [Dramatic gay pause, exhaling deeply to emphasize my feigned frustration.] "It's affecting my learning and causing severe headaches."

"Okay, Matthew, let's take a look."

Nurse Nancy asked me to stand on a yellow line approximately four feet from the supply closet. She asked me to face the standard eye chart on the outside of the door and read the fourth line.

I took a moment to absorb the white chart and the large black letters—despite being able to clearly make out every letter on the chart, I began slowly announcing the letters out loud; like Patrick Dempsey in the locker scene from *Can't Buy Me Love*.

By the time I was asked to read line six, E D F C Z P, I was completely (and clearly) making letters and words up; I even added numbers to sweeten the pot. Nurse Nancy's reaction was calm and concerned. "How long have you been having trouble with your vision, Matthew?"

"I guess about four months," I lied.

That evening my parents arrived to an answering machine message from the principal at Joseph Arnold Elementary school informing them that I had been struggling for several months with my vision, and upon an "alarming" visit with the school nurse, it had been established that Matthew needed glasses immediately.

My dad turned to me. "You're having trouble with your vision? Why didn't you say something to us?"

Always the professional, of course, I had dropped subtle hints at home, too: holding a box of cereal an inch from my face, struggling to identify words in the newspaper (I never read the newspaper prior to my love scheme), and groaning about headaches—all clues that went unnoticed.

"I don't know, I didn't think it was that big a deal." I was quick to reduce the *issue* in order to avoid being suspicious—unlike Mrs. Trevor, Nurse Nancy, and my principal, my parents knew exactly who I was and what I was capable of.

The following weekend my mom scheduled an appointment at the LensCrafters in our local mall. As if I were preparing for the Academy Awards, the night before my big examination I laid out the perfect outfit—something that would compliment the tortoise shell frames that I was planning to select. My not-too-vibrant faded Guess jeans (that I would peg) with an abstract (and ridiculously) over-the-top 90s rayon button down; the Drakkar Noir was placed alongside my white slouch-socks and pointy steal-front suede dress shoes. As if I'd forget to wear cologne to such an important event.

We arrived at the mall early, which gave us plenty of time to stop off at Gloria Jeans—the pre-Starbucks rage—and pick up a blended chocolate espresso drink. My favorite part was the chocolate-covered coffee bean on top of the pillow of whipped cream. I needed plenty of sugar, caffeine, and confidence for what was about to go down.

After filling out a pile of forms, my mom and I walked back into the examination room. I was suddenly overcome with a foreign feeling: Fear. I spent most of my early childhood in a constant state of make-believe; whether on the playground, dance class, or the cul-de-sac, I was always directing (bossing around) kids in magic shows, coaching classmates in school plays, and ordering neighbors to watch my performances in plays that I wrote myself. What I'm saying is—I was exceptional at marketing pretend.

Now, in the very REAL doctor's office (or as real as an exam room at the Del Amo Mall could be) I was going to *pretend* I needed glasses. This was the ultimate test of my acting abilities.

The first part of the exam was simple. I had to revisit the same eye exam chart from Nurse Nancy's office—this time I made smarter choices and I only pretended to miss every other letter. The optometrist didn't seem too concerned with my results. He smiled when I misidentified the final letter on the test and explained that I did very well.

Was this guy nuts? I missed more than half. I have never excelled at math (I'm more a words and facts kind of guy) but even I knew that fifty percent is bad. The follow up test was much more complicated, primarily because I didn't know what to expect, so I had no way of knowing how to cheat it.

The doctor instructed me to put my face against a masked device that looked more like an instrument of medieval torture. He asked me to look through the lens and just as he was explaining that I was going to feel slight pressure in my right eye—I was eye-raped with a shot of powerful air. "Ouch!" I jumped back two feet. I wasn't prepared to sacrifice so much pain for Hazuki, but Jeff was totally worth it.

Finally, I had to look through a kaleidoscope-esque contraption and properly distinguish colors and images. I decided to be honest on this test from fear of saying the wrong thing. The only control you have over the truth is to tell the truth whenever possible, even in the midst of a sophisticated scheme.

Once the tests were complete, the doctor (he was wearing a white lab coat so I'm pretty sure he was a doctor) shared the results with my parents. "Mr. and Mrs. Shaffer, Matthew did a very good job on his eye test. There's nothing serious, he did well and checked out normal on *most* of the examinations."

Most, that word was my saving grace! "Most?" my mom snapped.

"Well, Matthew struggles when reading words in close proximity, so I'm going to recommend a low prescription for reading glasses."

Sudden elation overcame my inner being. I was proud that my well-crafted plot had been a success! I was now ready to approach Hazuki as the four-eyed fifth grade dreamboat she'd always dreamed of.

First things first. I had to pick out a frame that would say, "Confident but not cocky," "fun but still hardworking," and "wise but not a square." After thirty minutes of browsing and trying on the different styles of frames, my mom and dad demanded that I make a choice. Unfortunately for me, they had limited my options to the more affordable LensCrafters frames, ruling out the $400.00 Ralph Lauren insta-popular glasses I had fallen in lust with. In the spirit of compromise, I found a pair of knock-off tortoise shell frames and called it a day.

With quality glasses, in about an hour I was ready to introduce the "new" me, at school. The second bell rang, alerting us that it was time to go to our homeroom class. I was outside with my classmates—Hazuki included—and not a single kid remarked on my spectacular specs. Back in Mrs. Trevor's room I was desperate for my peers to notice my new handicap; I raised my hand and adjusted the bridge of my glasses while asking an irrelevant question. After giving me a completely unsatisfactory answer, Mrs. Trevor took a moment, stared directly at my glasses and announced, "I'm delighted that you'll be able to focus a little more clearly now."

What? How vague is that reaction? I would have preferred that she call me Four Eyes!

During our second recess of the day (we had a lot more outdoor free time when I was a kid) I decided to go straight to the source. Hazuki played tetherball on our lunch break, so I knew she'd be doing death-drops on the high bars near the swings. I approached her as she was in her seventh rotation—in my closeted fifth-grade opinion Hazuki was destined for the Olympic team—and I waited for her to dismount.

I watched as she somersaulted to the ground and I made my move. "Hi Hazuki. Notice anything different?"

"No."

"Really?" I removed my streak-free glasses and picked up the bottom corner of my shirt to use as a glass cleaner.

I returned the already clean glasses back to my face and climbed on top of the medium bar (making sure that Hazuki could take her rightful place on the high bar next to me) and I started to warm-up my body by hanging upside down. Just like Kerri Strug, Hazuki remounted the high bar and we began our swing whips in unison. Foolishly, I attempted to do a double-death drop and as I was flying through mid-air I lost control and landed flat on my back, leaving just enough time to fart before the wind was knocked out of me.

Like an amateur musician rebounding from a bad set, I woke up in Nurse Nancy's office with the feeling of inferiority and shame; praying that the sound of my body hitting the dirt masked the sound of gas.

"Don't worry, passing gas is completely normal—especially when you get the wind knocked out of you."

Wonderful, if Nurse Nancy was already comforting me, the School-yard Express has certainly already spread the tale of the four-eyed farting boy.

I popped up and decided to face my fate. I walked back to Mrs. Trevor's class, where they were deep in discussion about how the legislative process works. I wished that I could have vetoed the last two hours of my life, but instead I held my head high and walked directly to my seat. As I approached the front row, I heard the faint sounds of armpit farts and muffled chuckling. Fartgate was going to linger for longer than the original smell, but I would bounce back.

After months of do-si-doing around Hazuki during our in-school square dancing lessons, our fifth grade class was finally ready to show our parents that we had successfully learned to co-exist with the opposite sex via the forum of a social dance where every instruction encourages you to "grab your partner and swing her around."

I spent most of our rehearsals trying to impress Hazuki, and instead all I'd done was become infatuated with her; the more I tried to impress her, the further she box-stepped away. Finally, I came right out and asked her if she liked me. Her answer was swift and unforgiving: "I like you as a friend, (whatever that means to a nine-year-old) but I only date boys with blond hair."

"Me too!" is what I wanted to say... Instead I walked away, crushed that my crush was over. I wasn't above putting Sun-In in my hair, but that wasn't on the cards for me until sixth grade (for Kristen White).

Like many things that would come to pass in my life, I committed to my cause and rode it out to the bitter end. In the end my pride was destroyed—and so were my eyes after wearing glasses that I didn't need for three months solid. I spent the next five months waiting for my eyes to refocus and when they finally did, they landed on an adorable Italian hockey player named Charlie Bonillio with deliciously curly, dark brown hair and tranquil blue eyes.

It's In the Jeans

A decade before the E! Channel launched the red carpet celebrity fashion strut into the spotlight; I was my mom, Julie's, personal stylist and all around shopping companion. We would spend hours combing the racks of the Macy's and Bloomingdale's petites sections for the perfect working woman's outfit. In no time at all, I acquired her taste for expensive fabrics, vibrant prints, and bold colors—adding an additional stop to the boy's Husky department in our already overbooked Saturday itinerary.

Swapping out Super Cuts (which my dad and sister far preferred) for the world of celebrity hairstylists, it was mom who taught me to indulge in the finer things in life. She once spent $400 to have José Eber hack into her enviously thick, shoulder-length brunette hair, leaving her with a butchered bob that was completely wrong for her face. The style was all the rage amongst the shoulder-pad clad women on TV in the 80s, but my mom was far too stunning for a flash in the pan fad. Had I not been on a Cub Scout retreat with my dad, I would have coaxed her towards a more classic cut.

By the early 90s, mom and I cultivated a meaningful allegiance with celebrity hairstylist Kimmy Rooney, who was the daughter of the legendary movie actor, Mickey Rooney. Tails of Mickey's torrid affairs, alleged abuse, and terrible parenting tactics would make my hair stand on end without product. It was in this high-end, Palos Verdes salon that I discovered how to gossip while appearing concerned, the proper way to apply mousse (just after the hair has been towel dried, but still damp), and I ascertained how practical the art of flattery could be. A woman always appreciates a complement, especially when she's spending upwards of $600 a month on her "natural beauty" to impress her wealthy husband who is surely cheating on her. I also learned an invaluable life lesson in my freshman year of high school that has stuck with me through adulthood: never let yourself get talked into ANYTHING.

It started out like any other trip to the posh boutique. Mom and I dashed over to Marci's Candy Shop to pick up Swedish Fish, Snow Caps, and chocolate covered peanuts. Adding another punch on my monthly membership card to the Chubby Closeted Kids Club. My mom could (and still does) devour junk food like most of Los Angeles consumes kale, and yet never gains a pound. Still, I caved to my cravings while trading dramatic stories with my mom about the events that unfolded during the week. My mom's youthful energy and playful personality made her an easy person to confide in. I never felt uncomfortable sharing my feelings.

While in the car we started talking about the characters in our favorite new show, *Beverly Hills 90210,* which was quickly becoming the replacement drama for the still juicy but not as fresh *Knots Landing.* I mentioned that I really liked Dylan McKay's hair, played by actor Luke Perry, and wanted Kimmy to cut my hair like his. Like every teenaged girl and closeted gay man, I had a huge crush on the Hollywood hottie. I couldn't admit it to myself then, although I'm sure my mom knew and totally accepted it, but getting my hair styled like his was my way of having him. When we arrived at the salon I revealed my desire to have Dylan's hairstyle and Kimmy smiled confidently and said, "Sure thing!"

I was hunched over the coffee table rummaging through a selection of beauty and lifestyle magazines when I saw Kimmy yank my mom into the dye-closet and whisper something in her ear. Were they on to me? I frantically ditched a copy of *The Enquirer*—which promised scandals from the set of *The Golden Girls*—and reached for the most masculine magazine I could find. *Newsweek* was hardly appropriate for a kid my age, but it was the only thing that didn't scream homo!

Kim sauntered over to collect me and casually mentioned that I would have to get a "body wave" in order to achieve Luke Perry's precious locks.

Uncomfortable with this developing information I asked, "A perm?"

"No. It's not a perm… it's a body wave," Kimmy replied.

"What's the difference?"

"A body wave is not as tight," she explained.

I took a sidebar with my mom to share my trepidation. My luxuriously luminous and ample head of hair was the one aspect of my life that I didn't loathe. Complete strangers would constantly stop me in shopping malls to gush endlessly over my marvelous mane. Not to brag, but my hair was so dazzling, that I was asked to model for a series of hairstyle books for a national beauty chain. Why was Kimmy so eager to chemically transform my magnificent mop?

"Mom, I don't want to get a perm. I'll be the laughing stock of high school."

"Matt, do you want to look like Luke Perry, or not?" My mom could sense my turmoil. I was dying to fit in, but my inner light was screaming to stand out.

Sensing trouble in HAIRadise, Kimmy slid in to close the deal.

"Matthew, I promise you that Luke Perry, Jason Priestley, and all of the teen heart throbs are getting body waves. It's the *only* way their hair can be styled the way you see it on TV."

Common sense told me that the kids at school would be cruel and oblivious to the current Hollywood trendsetters; but my ego said, "You'll finally be a heartthrob!"

"Well, if it's the only way… and they're all doing it… okay! Let's do it!" I was a pushover.

Both my mom and Kim's faces lit up like it was Christmas Day and I was a new Mercedes SL convertible parked in the driveway with a big red bow on it.

Against my intuition and everything I already knew about high school bullies, I sidestepped into the chair in front of Kimmy's mirror. I was the luxury vehicle—instead of a bow—Kim yanked strands of my hair and twisted the pink plastic rollers tight against my head until it was covered in strategic rows. Like a villain in a Disney movie, she formulated the concoction and applied the permanent solution to my head. I'll never forget the smell of betrayal.

Twenty minutes later my scalp was on fire and my eyes were watering. Kim expedited me to the rinse section and began urgently popping off the curlers, while rinsing away the chemicals—and my pride.

Back at her station, she maneuvered me into the chair before I could get a glance at my reflection. Using a circular brush and too much mousse she began manically blow-drying my hair. Finally, she stood back, pleased with her work, and revealed my TV star makeover.

There I was, the missing member of *New Kids On The Block*. Admittedly, I loved the look on me. It complemented my eyes and highlighted my high cheekbones. The fleeting exhilaration of pseudo stardom via a hair transformation was rapidly replaced with dread. The kids in my class would brand me forever as a faggot. Even at fourteen years old, I considered myself a talented actor, but no amount of Meisner technique could have disguised my sadness or kinky hair. I was longing to look like Luke Perry and was reprocessed into Gabrielle Carteris.

My anguish was so evident that Kimmy didn't even bother to try and pep me up. Wiping sympathetic tears away, my mom felt guilty and gushed over how handsome I was. She guaranteed that all of the girls at school were going to go crazy over my *Teen Beat* look.

My dad and sister were seated at the dinner table waiting for us when we barreled through the front door. Before he even said hello my dad automatically reacted, "Holy shit, what did you guys do now?" I burst into a grandiose fit of tears and ran to the bathroom, where I locked myself in and stared at the "camera ready" but dainty hair-DON'T.

My sister and dad continued laughing at me in the living room, while my mom whispered sternly to be sympathetic. Dealing with the critics eager to cast judgment rather than taking risks is something that my mom and I have in common. Dad and Shiree were content in their cotton-blend lifestyle and became amused and confused by anyone who preferred cashmere. Through bruised egos and frayed emotions, mom and I continued to brave the insults and ridicule, knowing that our self-expression and independence delivers a pleasure that far surpasses the anguish we've endured from less expressive individuals.

A knock at the bathroom door snapped me out of the mirror of confliction and into reality. My mom was ready with a master plan. She gathered her expensive hair products—the ones she kept hidden from the rest of the family—held my head under the bathroom sink and began working the pricey Paul Mitchell into a lather of suds and love. She rinsed and repeated this process at least four times, revealing that this would help relax the perm.

The following morning she rustled me out of bed early and helped me blow-dry my hair so that the curls would be less obvious to my friends and foes. We continued this morning ritual until my hair eventually surrendered its sassy stronghold on my locks. Three weeks felt like three years, but to my great fortune, not one person at school suspected a change in my appearance.

My mom has always been *that* person in my life who never questioned my motives or reacted to my impulses. Whether I woke up every morning and sat next to her vanity, watching intently as she applied her make-up before work, or whether I jumped into a pair of her pumps and practiced walking across her bedroom, she responded by validating my efforts: "You're better at that than I am!" making every moment seem normal.

Rather than trying to change my behaviors or reject my outlandish ideas, she celebrated our genetic similarities, teaching me how to capitalize on my passion and joy. Her colossal contribution to my adolescent development led me to seize every opportunity, be adventurous and unafraid to stand out from the crowd, and become the most valuable person in every job that I set out to do.

Above all else, she empowered me to stand up for myself in every circumstance. Including the time that my mom maxed out her credit card to invest in a pair of designer overalls that I was certain would secure my spot at the cool kids' table. When I showed up wearing the costly, fashion forward, "unisex" jeans on the same day as Lauren Terrell—the most popular girl in our class—mom motivated me to take action. She stood by me as I confronted the snobby GUESS® sales clerk, demanding my money back. It only took two hours, an assistant manager, and an emotionally charged outburst to close the deal. Yes, GQ declared that men *could* wear the en vogue farmer faux pas, but mom reminded me that when we fall victim to a marketing maneuver, it's okay to take a step back, regroup, and remember that who I am on the inside is more important than a magazine moment. Taking risks is always worth the ridicule when it aligns with our inner light; when the gamble doesn't pay off, courage and conviction will conquer all.

What Wood You Do?

In seventh grade, word spread that I was anal-retentive. I had no idea what it meant, but I automatically assumed that it had something to do with the tingling feelings I experienced while changing in the boys' locker room.

Concerned that my closest peers had discovered there was something wrong with me, I promptly dropped my recess activity—organizing other people's lockers—and ran directly to our dismal library. Crammed between the sparse book stacks I opened the outdated encyclopedia and hurriedly turned to the term: anal-retentive.

I read the comprehensive definition and I began compiling a mental list of all of the corresponding adjectives that defined anal retentiveness, also known as anally retentive or often abbreviated as anal. "Orderliness," "stubbornness," and "a compulsion for control"—were these really undesirable traits? Perhaps to an average teenager, but I was a focused artist on a mission. I was perfectly comfortable with these "leadership" qualities. I was slightly off-put by Freud's psychological connection to early pooping problems, but I shrugged his theories off as "too intellectual." At ease that my friends were labeling me as a bossy overachiever and not a homo, I headed to my fourth period wood shop class.

Mr. McKenny was our no-nonsense, never-crack-a-smile wood shop teacher. Stalky not fat, his posture was erect and authoritative. He stuck me as the type of man who spent his nights polishing his massive gun collection and his weekends reenacting the Civil War. His hair was receding in the middle and fuzzy on the sides—imagine Sidney

Poitier minus the talent, charm, and the OSCAR. He would demand attention by smacking a yardstick on mounds of well organized but overrun manuals that sat atop his solid oak desk.

His list of rules and safety regulations was longer than the blade on the hacksaw that hung off the side of his desk, which he claimed he would use on a textbook if he caught us using his class for a free study period, rather than "focusing on the wood." He took wood shop very seriously—rightfully so; the truth is that 40 seventh graders had unsupervised access to table saws, drill presses, torches, band saws, and dozens of poisonous chemicals.

At the beginning of each semester, Mr. McKenny selected one industrious student to act as the foreman in order to help monitor the potential catastrophes that lurked in every corner. The job title came with an automatic grade bump. If you were receiving a "B" in the class, you'd advance with an "A." The duties included maintaining structure, inspecting projects, anticipating potential accidents, and most importantly, calling the five-minute warning to ensure that our classroom was completely spotless before we left for lunch each day. Mr. McKenny was a stickler for an immaculate work environment and made it very clear that whomever he chose for the coveted role would be responsible for the condition of the classroom at all times. It was a burden that only a strong know-it-all with OCD could accept. When he stated to the entire class as fact: "Mr. Shaffer, you're outgoing and anal-retentive. Would you like the job?" Wow. Even the teachers had jumped on the anal attack! Fine—I happily accepted the undertaking.

Woodshop was different from our other classes. We didn't learn from standard textbooks and our grades relied heavily on our craftsmanship and creativity. It was labeled as an "elective class", which was funny, because every seventh grader was required to take it in order to advance to eighth grade. Subsequently, an air of resentment and burnt wood shavings filled the oversized classroom. It didn't help that the class came right before our lunch period, so most of us were starving while operating heavy machinery.

The first few weeks of class we studied the equipment and familiarized ourselves with the varieties of wood, plastic, and aluminum. Once we could successfully identify a hard wood from a soft wood and discriminate between a metal cutter and a wood saw, we proceeded to sanding and stains. From there we learned how to make patterns and eventually we developed the ability to use a hacksaw and make crappy doorstoppers or paperweights. Over time, we were given the space to make supervised cuts on the bigger saws, which led to shabby holiday gifts that our parents would no doubt hide in the basement.

At first, my role as foreman was fairly straightforward. I had to bully a few kids into returning the equipment in a timely manner, pick up the excess scrap wood around their tables, and yell when someone would run with a pair of scissors; nothing out of the ordinary.

But as soon as the tools were turned on, the power went to my head. Suddenly I found myself lurking over the shoulders of my comrades. The more adventurous our projects got, the more involved our cleanup process became. Five minutes before our bell, I would blow a whistle, which I swiped from my dad's referee bag, to alert the class that it was time to wrap up. It was an effective way to get everyone's attention over the ear-piercing machinery. My woodworking friends felt otherwise.

Over the course of the semester, I noticed that fewer kids were picking up after themselves. They'd discovered that I would trail them, picking up any debris left behind, in order to maintain my contract (and good standing name) with Mr. McKenny. I also wanted to get to my lunch on time.

Soon, the entire class was ignoring my warnings and laughing at my empty threats. They knew that only Mr. McKenny had the authority to keep kids after school, and he would never back me up so I was left eating sawdust.

Several of my teachers, mentors, and my parents cautioned that I had unusually high standards for a middle school student, which might not win popularity votes. I accepted that my work ethic, take-charge personality, and discipline was an asset in my growth as an artist—but left kids my age feeling incompetent, lazy, and insecure. I struggled not to let their name-calling and mocking nature get under my skin. Despite my generally sunny disposition, I am human; eventually we all have our breaking point.

My Balsa tree branch finally snapped on what began like an ordinary Thursday morning. I rehearsed choreography on my walk to school, finished my homework (from the night before) during first period English, gorged on donuts that I bought from the bake sale, and gossiped during recess with my girlfriends. Once I reached shop class I was prepared—thanks to the aforementioned gabfest—for our WOOD-be substitute teacher.

Unless you grew up on a different planet or never maneuvered through middle school, you understand that a substitute teacher means one thing: total chaos. Unlike many Southern California schools (in deep denial), Calle Mayor Middle School recognized that their overly entitled and privileged students were highly unlikely to behave for a sub and therefore implemented a "busy work only" policy. Rather than expecting the temporary teacher to *teach* us something from our curriculum, they handed out Xeroxed copies of crossword puzzles, word searches, and vocabulary drills.

I entered the classroom and immediately observed that none of my classmates were sitting in their assigned seats—let the games begin. I walked over to introduce myself to our substitute, Mr. ProveThemWrong, and explained my role as foreman. I fashioned myself as more of a teacher's confidant than a student, so I made sure to clue him in on the assigned seating and pointed him toward the filing cabinet full of ditto copied busy work.

"Class as usual today, ladies and gentlemen, and I'm not afraid to hand out detention, so please find your way to the pine that belongs to your behind," he projected at the top of his lungs, while selling me out about the musical chairs.

I absorbed the glares and whispers as I pulled the ax from my back and took my seat.

"Why do you always have to be such a goody-goody?" "Are you addicted to kissing ass?" "Do you even know how to be *normal*?" And my personal favorite… "You're such a faggot—you can't have fun unless you're being butt raped." These were just a few of the hateful words that my *friends* felt the need to express in between sanding and varnishing their shitty wood sticks.

I watched the clock slowly tick while my peers went out of their way to leave the classroom in total disarray. Breaking every rule, they took tools out without returning them, flicked scraps of wood from table to table like they were mini footballs, opened jars of chemical bonding agents they didn't even use, and left dirty paint brushes dripping off the sides of workstations. My dad is a plumbing contractor and I've seen abandoned construction sites with less debris. Not even all of the work-for-hires waiting in the parking lot at Home Depot could tackle this disaster zone. I'm supposed to ask my peers to clean this up in five minutes? Absolutely KNOT!

With fifteen minutes of class remaining, I blew my whistle. Several of the more understanding kids (mainly low-level nerds who kept to themselves) contributed to the clean up efforts; everyone else stood still.

First, I tried to reason with everyone, "Come on guys, I get it… but we can't leave here until the room is clean." Crickets.

"Seriously, aren't you all hungry? If this space isn't up to Mr. McKenny's standards, you know we'll be in trouble." Still nothing. It dawned on me that they didn't care—they weren't responsible—they were leaving as soon as the bell rang.

I was furious. My face was flushed. I could feel my heartbeat in my cheeks as I stormed around the room with my arms in the air. Screaming at the top of my lungs while picking up everyone's discarded materials. At one point, I took my arm (like a scene in a romantic comedy when the characters are going to have spontaneous sex on a countertop) and I swept all of the wood and trash onto the floor. My peers watched with joy and delight as I paced around the shop with a push broom like a chainsaw cutting through a Christmas tree, until finally all that remained was a tiny opened jar of paint thinner.

I walked toward the desk where the solvent sat and demanded, "WHO USED THIS?" No answer—no surprise. Raging, I reached for the paintbrush from the potent, thin mixture. As I lifted the handle from the container the bristles from the synthetic brush caught the edge of the jar and a tsunami of poison engulfed my face.

My eyes had been introduced to a sea of toxic chemicals that would no doubt begin eating away at my retinas, rendering me permanently blind. In every direction—through the inflamed slits that were my eyelids—I saw my peers pointing and laughing. Not a single classmate volunteered to help me. Granted, I'd been a total timber tyrant for the better part of a semester, but were they really just going to stand there and watch me go visionless?

I ran past my best friend Tommy, who stood on the fence of popularity and sympathy—Et tu, Brute? Like a *Milli Vanilli* fan that had just discovered the pop duo's lip sync lie, I ran in frenzy down the open-aired hallways of Calle Mayor Middle School. Straight past the secretary and into the nurse's office (where soon I, too, would have my very own punch card) and screamed at the top of my lungs: "I'm going blind!"

Thankfully, Nurse Nancy's office was unoccupied and she was swift to react. Utilizing her soothing voice to extract the facts of my melodramatic mishap, she prepared the eye-flushing station, which was readily on deck.

In a routine manner, she walked me over to a unit near the sink that looked like a drinking fountain; only instead of a spout for water there were two green plastic cylinders that looked like upside-down bells. She instructed me to lean forward and place my eyes over the circular spouts. She explained that it was important that I hold my eyes open with my hands for fifteen minutes to ensure that all of the dangerous chemicals are flushed away.

As she pumped the lever to begin the flow of solvent she exclaimed in a happy tone, "I've never had to use this station before!" After the less than comforting declaration, the first splash of fluid doused my eyes. Instantly they stopped burning and I started to relax. Three minutes into the baptism, and it felt like my eyes were going to drown. Similar to opening your eyes under water in an over chlorinated pool, I could make out fuzzy images, but I still wasn't certain I would regain full vision. During the following twelve minutes, the warm eyewash felt like a reinvigorating massage for my eyeballs. Then, the moment of truth. Nurse Nancy helped me to a chair and my eyes were reborn!

She took a moment to examine my eyes (if you're keeping track, this was a familiar circumstance for both of us) and she determined that no permanent damage had been done. In an effort to avoid any light sensitivity, she placed a gauze bandage over each eye and asked me to lie down on the examination table, where I stayed for the remainder of the afternoon.

When the bell rang signaling the end of the school day, I stayed hidden in the nurse's office until I was certain that all of my peers had left. Not one of them checked in on me following the incident. The last yellow bus cleared the parking lot and I cautiously made my exit through the back door normally reserved for administration and hall monitors only.

My house was only three blocks from school but the ordinarily short walk felt like an epic trek as I rehashed the events of the day over and over again in my head. Why was I such a freak? How could I be so careless with a dangerous chemical? Why didn't any of my friends help me?

I was so resentful that I skipped my after-school dance and acting classes, and locked myself in my bedroom. My eyes felt normal, but I couldn't see clearly; my heart was heavy with disappointment. I couldn't understand why I got so exasperated with the other kids in my class for not participating in the clean-up efforts, and worse, why they would mock me in the midst of doing their jobs. Suddenly a word popped into my head: selfishness. It was selfish of them to take advantage of the fact that I would always clean up their messes and it was selfish of me to impose my own compulsions on a group of seventh graders who probably didn't even make their own bed, comb their own hair, or decide what they were going to wear each day.

The following morning I returned to school with a new perspective. When the bell rang for fourth period I reported directly to woodshop, where I found Mr. McKenny back behind his desk. I approached him without raising my hand—a blatant violation of his rigid rules—and I offered my resignation as foreman. He took a moment before responding with a patronizing tone, "I heard things got a little out of control. I expected more from you." Like most of my friends who had come to know my personality, I'm sure he anticipated a big reaction; instead I simply grinned and returned to my seat.

Before I even reached my table, Mr. McKenny stood up and announced a new foreman. My peers avoided eye contact with me for the rest of the period.

When the newly appointed foreman called "clean up" five minutes before the end of class, I sat motionless at my workstation and didn't lift a finger. I watched as the rest of my class frantically swept up sawdust, wiped down the machines, and returned tools to the toolbox. All around me, my subordinates worked together to restore the luster of our workspace. My silent protest spoke just as loud as their wordless apology.

Notwithstanding my feelings for a sterilized and structured work environment, I disengaged from the cleaning duties for the rest of the semester. If teachers and students were so ardent and deliberate to mock my industrious work ethics, I was equipped to show them how my anal-retentive decorum benefitted me. At once order was renewed in my universe. The pressure from my blistering perfectionism was relieved as soon as I pulled out a small sliver of my obsessive-compulsive disorder.

Drama Queen

Transitioning from a state-of-the-art performing arts high school on a palm tree lined campus in Southern California, to a public high school in a rural area of Colorado overrun by dairy farms, cement plants, and the largest cluster of prisons in the state, promised to be more "rocky" than "mountain high".

I was trading the fame, fashion, and flair of Hollywood for Wrangler jeans, cans of Copenhagen, and cruising Main Street. My senior class at Florence High School had less than one hundred students; most had no interest in anything other than rodeos and the Denver Broncos. I managed to keep my cool for the first few weeks of school, slowly seeking out any other kids who stood out. If they wore anything that wasn't branded (literally) or threw in an occasional pop song between country calamities on their mix-tapes, I immediately befriended them.

By the end of the first semester I had assembled a group of eclectic gypsies who strayed from the jocks, the nerds, and the cheerleaders to form a clique of culture, bad skin, and risky—albeit poor—choices in wardrobe.

My next objective was to start a Drama Club. I quickly realized this was going to be more challenging than convincing a cowboy to swap out his hat for hair products, especially because the only organization anyone in the town actually joined was the 4H Club.

All school sanctioned clubs and organizations had to be supervised by a teacher and I was desperate to find my ideal candidate. A renegade who possessed the ability to persuade the principal when needed and fend off other teachers who would try to steal our rehearsal space; the gym was a hot commodity. This pawn would be present at all of our functions, but turn a blind eye to the zany antics of high school drama dorks. A leader to take charge when members of the club got caught up in the *drama* that naturally ensues in a Drama Club but remain on the sidelines while I was directing. We needed a former theater geek.

Fate intervened when I met Mrs. Riggs a few weeks earlier. Though she was actually my sister's freshman English teacher, I came to know Mrs. Riggs after a brief encounter during a school assembly. I complemented the courageous choice of color in her wardrobe (like any closeted teen would) and she blushed as she thanked me and told me that she was not afraid of style.

An instant admiration and mutual respect was formed, because neither of us was shy about living our lives out loud. Once we discovered that she also had to maneuver around the temperate of my adorable yet sometimes complicated sister—we became instant BFF's.

Mrs. Riggs was young compared to all of the other teachers. She was boisterous, outgoing, and loved all things theater, dance, and pop culture. She stood tall and confident with dark brown hair, porcelain skin, and animated brown eyes. What I hadn't discovered yet, is that Mrs. Riggs had a set of pipes and was ready to serenade our school with Betty Buckley fabulousness.

Knowing that she ate alone in her classroom, I approached her in the middle of our lunch period to make my plea. When I arrived she appeared to be in deep thought while eating a salad from a Tupperware container proving both healthy and practical; I was really falling for Mrs. Riggs.

I could see her eyes light up during my passionate fifteen-minute monologue, excerpts of which may have been lifted from *Clueless*. When I finally finished my *performance* Mrs. Riggs stood up from behind her desk, walked around to face me head on, and gave me a big hug.

"I'm in!"

In order to form a club we needed to find twenty students willing to sacrifice their free time to learn lines and play pretend, which in high school, was harder than I thought it would be. Our mission was to find likeminded students who were eager to share their artistic side; an almost impossible task in a community where hunting was equally regarded as a hobby, sport, and mandated rite of passage. I had confidence that I could entice the outcasts, closet-cases (like myself), and the eccentrics to abandon one lunch period a week to join forces in a display of thespian flair.

I started the process by reaching out to my campus crew, whom I hung out with regularly. Well adjusted teenagers who excelled academically but had accepted that they had no desire to belong to an athletics team or cling to a group of kids in order to feel important, and above all—they had already started planning their exit strategy from small town U.S.A.

Though skeptical at first, when I informed them that we would be taking our productions "on the road" during school hours, they jumped on board. From there I managed to convince a group of the not-so-popular students that they would have protection against the jocks if we joined forces; obviously an easy sell. Finally, I had to bring out the heavy artillery for the independently strong rebels like the Goths and "hipsters" (before we knew to label them as such). Considering most of them dyed their hair and wore clothing that looked more like costumes, I didn't think this was such a farfetched idea. I sealed the deal when I assured them that this would add a layer of intrigue and fuel them with freshly inspired fodder for when they attended their coffeehouse poetry jam sessions.

With our band of misfits now perfectly cast it was time for the action. It was clear to everyone involved that I would assume the role of Drama Club President. Given that I was the biggest diva in the group I decided to appoint myself the Vice President and Treasurer of the club—no doubt violating the official club election rules—but we had a laundry list of drudgery to get done and we didn't have time to waste on technicalities.

Like my designer jeans, salon quality hair products, and growing addiction to Starbucks, mounting a play is expensive and we needed cash. During our first meeting I suggested that we sell cotton candy at all of the athletic events. A job that had been abandoned by the girls' gymnastics team when their coach discovered that they were eating more than they were selling. My sister was on the team and offered up the insider information as long as I promised her an endless supply of the caloric confection. Their weight gain was a financial loss for them, but a sweet treat for us!

Pink pillows of candy clouds lined our coffer with the revenue stream we needed to begin pre-production on our play. Mrs. Riggs had gone out of her way to preselect several popular plays that were making the rounds on the high school drama circuit. While I appreciated her with eagerness to produce a play, I challenged her choice in content. First, *Romeo and Juliet*. The tone was perfectly suited for our town's ongoing feud between the churchgoing white-collar workers and the bar squatting blue-collar laborers. I feared the irony would be lost on their children. Plus, most of our club struggled to speak in full sentences, so I didn't think they would fare well with iambic pentameter. Next she suggested *Our Town*. Surely I would have delivered a crowd pleasing performance as the *Stage Director*, but the content of the play itself would have come across more like a city council meeting than a theatrical event. Finally, there was *Steel Magnolias*. I loved the movie. Nearly every line is quotable—including the ones Julia Roberts butchers—but the play is a female driven story with only five characters; none of whom are men. Unless the town was ready for me to channel my inner Dustin Hoffman a la *Tootsie*, "Drink your juice, Mrs. Riggs" because the beauty shop is closed!

Never one to arrive anywhere without ammunition (I might have been new to this country community, but I understood survival of the fittest), I had also prepared a selection of works to pitch to our group. Perhaps with more of an agenda, I was sure to include the "throwaway plays" which included *Uncle Vanya*—too long, and *Angels In America*—too gay; leaving only room for my own brainchild: *A Tribute To Shel Silverstein*. The concept was based on a remarkable hybrid of Dr. Seuss stories that were weaved together in a seamless twenty-minute performance during a theater competition that I attended in high school years before the tragedy, known as *Seussical The Musical.*

The formula was perfect for a high school setting. Mrs. Riggs and I incorporated sixteen of Shel's most popular poems and added short transitions and interstitials. The dialogue rhymed, making it easier for our less-trained actors to memorize the script, and the stories were so over-the-top that we could use homemade props and costumes to convey a whimsical tone and save on production costs. My primary objective was to position the Drama Club with enough clout and cash to produce a musical in the spring.

Score one for the duo of Riggs and Shaffer! *A Tribute To Shel Silverstein* was a massive success in our tiny community. We performed every weekend and some weeknights throughout the months of November and December. Our show was being requested by every senior center, nursing home, elementary school, and ribbon cutting across the county. We even made the local paper—twice! If you had blue hair, an occasional *accident* in your pants, or wore overalls, you knew who we were.

Mrs. Riggs and I knew that we had a limited window to capitalize on our big time buzz. We also confirmed that the bizarre mix of characters that joined forces to populate our Drama club actually had the chops to pull off something grandiose.

Enter Stage Left: me holding a revised version of *Cats* entitled *Mad Cats*. My dream show was still on Broadway, making it impossible to secure the rights. *Feline, fearless, faithful, and true*—for two weeks straight, I spent every evening and most of my fifth period Spanish classes adapting the lyrics and *script*. I use the word "script" loosely; even then I understood that Andrew Lloyd Webber's work was less about the lyrics and more about the melodies—er—dancing? Let's not get snobby about it. We all agree that it proved entertaining enough to sustain Broadway audiences for decades.

Following our holiday break, I passed out the abridged copies of our spring production. Cautious at first, my peers were not as elated about the MEOWsical selection as I had hoped.

I am remarkable at convincing people to do what I want. Generally because they get tired of hearing me talk and just give in. Such was the case with *Mad Cats*. Once I was finished describing our interactive set, special effects (including a fog machine I secured from a local Halloween fanatic), and the opportunity to tease the audience as we danced past their seats, I had the entire cast eating the catnip out of my hands. Because… *Jellicles can and Jellicles do, Jellicles do and Jellicles can, Jellicles can and Jellicles do…* You get the message—and so did Broadway, for 18 years.

Collectively, we the drama people, decided to add another day to our pre-production schedule, bringing us together three times a week. Those of us who really took our craft seriously decided to meet on the weekends, too. A production of this magnitude required attention to detail.

Discarded mattresses, mounds of trash bags filled with bunched up newspapers, tires, and worn furniture—anything we could gather from junkyards, backyards, or off curbs on the way to school—became the foundation for our set. With daring artistry, we took cans of spray paint and blasted the walls with phrases like, "Keep Out", "No Dogs Allowed", and my personal favorite, "Kool Katz". By the end of the second week our entire multipurpose performing arts center, which was really just the old gymnasium covered in carpeted risers, was transformed into the alley of an off-off-off-off-off-off Broadway version of *Cats*.

Time to tackle the creative agenda. Rigorous improvisational movement exercises followed the traditional singing, dancing, and acting cuts that took place during our audition process. After an hour of rubbing our bodies against one another and using our mouths to send balls of yarn back and forth across the stage, Mrs. Riggs and I had seen enough. For lack of stronger talent, I received the coveted part of *Mr. Mistoffelees* and Mrs. Riggs was the only suitable candidate for *Grizabella, the Glamour Cat*.

In order to give everyone plenty of time to practice the dance steps we jumped into the major musical numbers first. It turns out I'm gifted at choreographing for non-dancers. Their lack of technical training provides the perfect canvas for my practical story driven movement. Where a studied dancer might challenge my conceptualization, a novice "actor-who-moves" is motivated by my pedestrian qualities. It was in these early productions that I ascertained the skill to categorize those who can dance, those who can learn, and those who can stand in the background with a prop. Anyone who couldn't kick-ball-change on the count was separated from the litter and given an oversized beach ball. With enough glitter on the costumes, gelled lights, trampolines, and circular running patterns, everything looked stunning.

Once the choreography was set, Mrs. Riggs dedicated her talents to coaching the vocal and acting rehearsals. Because there was very little dialogue, she was able to spend most of her energy drilling the music over and over again. After several weeks of scaling the walls, the cast was finally singing in purrrrfect harmonies. Mrs. Riggs and I had masterfully morphed our gym into a junkyard and our cast into cats. In order to boost sales, we decided to invite the entire school to an informal in-school run of the first act of our show during fourth period.

By lunch, we were the cat's meow and sold out all six performances by the end of the week.

Opening night was everything I dreamed it would be. The crowd gathered in anticipation outside the auditorium doors. Inside, the cast and crew scurried around making last minute adjustments to the costumes and scenery. I was busy reviewing the lighting and music cues and making sure that our fog machine had plenty of fluid to keep the stage adequately hazed, ensuring the audience would receive the proper alley cat vibe.

Suddenly my heart sank. Moments before we opened the house, it dawned on me that I had spent so much of my time and energy making sure that the cast knew their choreography, staging, lines, and music that I never thought to check in with Mrs. Riggs regarding her performance. Should it have concerned me that we skipped her part in every tech rehearsal and run-through? Whenever we'd get to her part she'd say, "I want it to be a surprise for you!" It made sense in the moment. She seemed qualified for the job, but now, with the entire town in attendance, I was panicking. My name was all over the program: *Mad Cats*, adapted by Matthew Shaffer, co-directed by Matthew Shaffer, choreographed by Matthew Shaffer, starring Matthew Shaffer as Mr. Mistoffelees. Was my entire reputation as a writer/director/choreographer/actor going to be tarnished so early in my career? Too late to worry now, it was show time.

The lights faded to black and the *Overture* began. Jumping, twirling, and circling around, the cast owned the stage with feline grace and confidence. In every direction I witnessed a sense of pride and accomplishment—a group of unlikely high school students united to form a club that dedicated our precious afterschool hours to playing make-believe. The moment of truth came in the second act shortly after I had successfully finished my big dance solo, which included nailing 32 fouetté pirouettes in a row (not an easy task to do on carpeted risers I might add), and it was time for Mrs. Riggs to make her Florence High School debut.

From behind a heap of junk piled high stage right, *Grizabella* made her slow entrance to center stage. Mustering every ounce of anguish, regret, and disappointment that all high school English teachers must feel at some point in their career, Mrs. Riggs embodied the washed up "Glamour Cat". The first cord of *Memory* was played and she raised her head to meet the light, which caught her melancholy expression as she sang her first note. The exquisite balance of her tender restraint and confident belt, while expressing the devastating truth of the song, left no doubt in anyone's mind who the star of our show was.

I'd spent the entire year foolishly believing that I was in charge. With the subtlety and beauty that only a truly collaborative artist can spare, Mrs. Riggs generously allowed me to gleam—and in doing so—she was the one who shone the brightest in the end. Mrs. Riggs had become my Drama Queen!

Whether it was my triumphant turn as an acrobatic cat, the fact that I was the only president to make money for a school organized club, or my successful push to have the Drama Club transitioned into a legitimate class the following school year, the administration was so impressed that they started a scholarship in my name.

Each year, beginning with me, one graduating senior received the Matthew Shaffer Drama Scholarship toward a university or professional training institute of their choice. Success! I'd left my mark in the litter box at Florence High School. Over and above, I cultivated my collaborative spirit, polished my prowess as producer, and triumphed over my fear of wearing tights in public. Sadly, shortly after Mrs. Riggs' departure, they cut the acting class and subsequently the scholarship in my name. I guess not all cats have 9 lives.

AOL Chat Room

In 1996, *Ace Of Base* was my go to group, I had a standing date with *Friends* on Thursday nights, and teenagers everywhere were discovering illicit and exquisite private clubs known as AOL chat rooms. I was one of the fortunate teenagers to have an inside track to the dial-up Internet, thanks to my WAY-ahead-of-her-time friend, Leah.

Like me, Leah wasn't afraid to raise eyebrows in unconventional ways. Her long, lean, and well-defined physique housed a Mensa mind and a dry—but hilarious—personality. Leah's adventurous blue eyes sparkled when she spoke about her plans after high school—another reason we connected—she *had* plans for her life after high school. She possessed that strange and winning combination of athlete and MATHlete. Leah broke the Colorado state record for running the fastest mile, beating out all of the males and females who crawled in her way. In the same week, she claimed victory over the undefeated reigning state chess opponent, and was awarded full scholarships to several prestigious universities.

When she wasn't fully committed to overachieving, she liked to hang out with me. Probably because we shared the same ludicrous drive to dominate at everything we do, and I made her laugh.

Leah's house was across the street from our high school and became the ideal spot for us to escape the confines of unpleasant lunch period banter. Mostly, we spent our time talking about the things that roused us. She lectured me on the importance of recycling, while gathering trash for her compost heap. I repurposed anecdotal teenage quotes from the movie *Clueless*. Leah preached that greenhouse gases were destroying our Ozone. I proclaimed the power of applying SPF and stressed a daily skin care regiment. She rambled on about marine biology with zest and confidence, while I recited Shakespeare.

Midway through our senior year, Leah's father invested significantly towards her future, buying her a Windows based PC. Four boxes, a cluster of cords, and team of techies with trifocals later, we could *finally* use the hundreds of CD's that America Online sent each month for something other than a coaster. With over 300 hours of free AOL dial-up now at our disposal, things were about to get wild. CuurrssshhhhhhhhhhRRRRRIIIIIINNnnnn BBBeeeeePPppppppCCUUUURrrrshhh… "Welcome. You've got mail!"

Waiting for those beautiful words was often torture. We only had 45 minutes before we'd have to go back for fifth period Spanish and the information super highway had more traffic than the 405 Freeway. Connecting to AOL often took several unsuccessful attempts and switching between four different phone numbers until finally we were granted access to the exclusive and anonymous chat rooms.

I sat eagerly next to Leah as she typed in a series of codes that would lead us deeper into the swampland of the web. "Men seeking young women." "Men seeking hot chicks." "Men seeking men." "Men seeking married women." "Men seeking married men." There was no doubt a slew of desperate, lonely, men sitting in the obscurity of their basements across America, hunting for innocent young prey.

I was ready to be captured, or at least ravished by sexually charged words that I would later fantasize about in the security of my bedroom.

Leah had several pseudo screen names that we would switch between while waiting for replies from repugnant, horny men. We had our favorites saved on a special list. Those guys who would start off sweet and affectionate and then go Jeffrey Dahmer on us. It was strange that these monsters felt so comfortable sharing their twisted delusions with random strangers. Then again, they were getting aroused exchanging sex chats with (mostly) virginal children pretending to be eager young women. Perhaps they suspected that and it added a layer of titillation to their perverted power trip.

<MuscleMan1969>

Hey beautiful. How are you today?

<ColoradoQT> (One of our screen names)
Sad.

<MuscleMan1969>
Why so sad?

<ColoradoQT>
I failed my Algebra exam. Getting a D in the class.
Dad is going to take away my computer.

<MuscleMan1969>
NOOO. I need your sweet pussy.

<ColoradoQT>
I know baby. I need your rock hard dick inside me
now.

<MuscleMan1969>
I'm throwing you down on my bed right now.

<ColoradoQT>
Be gentle.

<MuscleMan1969>
I thought you liked it rough?

<ColoradoQT>
I'm still sore from our last time. : (

<MuscleMan1969>
This is going to hurt then. ;) My massive cock is
throbbing right now. Take a deep breath.

AOL Voiceover: "Goodbye"

With a swift kick to the crotch, the Internet gods had logged us off—just as we were getting turned on. Our online role-play exploration continued for several weeks until Leah asked the question that I had avoided having to admit out loud.

"Why don't you ever want to pretend to be the man in these chat rooms and go after girls?"

I responded in my mind first: "Because it's more exhilarating to get a man off, than think about a woman's vagina."

I was a senior in high school and still a virgin. I walked around professing that I was too invested in my training as a dancer to commit to a relationship. Throughout middle school and into high school I'd had a few girlfriends for appearance's sake. Beards, before I even knew that a beard could be more than just hair on a man's face, but we never went further than second base. I was more interested in picking up a hotdog at the concession stand than swinging my bat around the turf hoping for a grand slam.

Not one of the girls I dated ever produced that indescribably intoxicating euphoria that starts in your gut and works its way to every nerve ending in your body. The men online gave me the permission to talk dirty, the ability to feel sexual, the mental images to satisfy my cravings later, and the swagger to walk back to fifth period Spanish with wet pants (just like all of the other boys in my class). The nasty, primal urges from anonymous male chat rooms *finally* made me feel like a normal dude.

I couldn't admit this to Leah, so I smiled and said, "I could never talk to a girl like that!" She smiled and said, "*That's* why I love you."

That was the last time we signed on to an AOL Chat room. I think we both realized we'd reached our climax.

Shit Happens

We all have unexplainable phobias; mine is shitting in public places. Considering the extreme case of early-onset OCD, the sandbox in my backyard was hardly a suitable place to drop a BM. Try telling that to my parents, who not so lovingly locked us outside so that they could focus on whatever moms and dads do in the middle of a Saturday morning. After several minutes of hollering and banging at the sliding glass doors which separated five-year-old me from our clean porcelain potty—I had to take matters into my own hands before they ended up in my pants. Despite my modest manners in all things bathroom related (it was and remains the only place in my life where I'm shy) I had no other option, it was time to go—with or without my parents' help.

I was both resourceful and swift to take action. In this case, I ran over to the 6 x 6 trench of sand that my dad had painstakingly sectioned off with abandoned railroad ties earlier that summer. I discarded my pants and stepped up onto the highest of the uneven logs that segregated the sand from the sea of grass. Striking a squatting stance (which I now identify as "Chair pose" thanks to years of yoga) I expelled my waste similar to the way a cement truck pours concrete. The shame of staring down at the King-sized crap combined with the look of intrigue and disgust on my sister's face as she witnessed the deposit became the foundation for my fear of public pooping.

* * *

No longer excited to shop in the husky section at Macy's or continue to be affectionately identified as Fat-Matt by "friends", I decided to develop an eating disorder at the end of my seventh grade year. I was old enough to understand that I was eating my feelings, but wasn't sure how to end my love affair with anything dipped in a trough full of ranch dressing. The zesty, creamy dip was the culinary cure for all of my problems; and as a 4' 9" thirteen-year-old boy with a size thirty-six inch waist, a flair for the arts, and a voice that was still a soprano—I needed all of the sauce I could get my soft, pudgy hands on.

On my way home from a particularly terrible day at school, on which several of my insecure classmates had found a way to gay bash and fat shame me at the same time, I realized it was time to take action. My passion for dance and the performing arts was in full production mode, which obviously intimidated the haters. I concluded that if I was focused enough to balance my free time between hours of dance, acting, and vocal classes while maintaining a 3.8 GPA—I could find the discipline to control my relationship with food.

My decrease in consumption started off casually. I'd seen enough after-school specials to understand that I did not want to draw attention to my disorder; instead I proactively declared to my parents and dance teachers that I was going on a strict diet. I started counting calories (long before there was an app) and significantly reduced the amount of food I was eating.

Three weeks into my "healthier" lifestyle, I was down ten pounds and two pant sizes; this should have been a red flag to anyone who understands survival, but instead family and friends alike praised my sudden transformation. The validation and attention led me on the fast track to anorexia where portion control meant not eating. Added bonus: counting calories is easier when there's nothing to count.

For several weeks I maintained a regular schedule of not eating while dancing six hours a day. It was only a matter of time before the stomach cramps became harder to bear than watching reruns of *The Facts of Life*. Worse, my toilette hadn't seen the number two in over three weeks. Ask any doctor and they'll confirm, that is not a good thing.

On the one hand, I looked exactly how I'd always imagined I should as an aspiring dancer: extremely thin. My body no longer felt the rush of adrenaline that starving your body can provide in small doses, and had transitioned into actual starvation.

When I could no longer disguise the way my small intestine had waged on my body, I decided I had to say something. But how do you tell your parents you've been deliberately starving yourself because you're tired of getting fat-shamed for having B-cup boobs that bounce around during dance class?

I concluded that the only way out of this was to act like I had a stomachache and beg for the "pink stuff".

"Pepto-Bismol?" My dad asked.

"Yes, I think that will make me feel better."

"Well tell me this, do you have to poop, or do you have diarrhea?"

"Dad, why does it matter? Just give me some of the Pepto-Bismol so I can feel better! I don't really want to talk about my poop with you."

"Son, it's important because Pepto-Bismol can cause constipation, so if you're already constipated, we'll need something else."

"Oh, in that case, get me something else!"

This conversation continued for what felt like days, until finally he gave me some Imodium—and I waited. Hours passed, nothing. NO movement. Now in full panic mode, I began to cry out of frustration; yet another attempt to be normal (or at least look normal) had backfired and my bowels were paying the consequences.

With no other options, I decided to divulge the scandal to my parents. I could not process their lack of concern. Wouldn't most parents be (at the very least) mildly panicked? I know that "The Seaver's" staged an intervention when they discovered their daughter "Carol's" anorexia on an episode of *Growing Pains*. Sure, it was a TV family—and it may have been Tracey Gold (the actress who played Carol Seaver) who had the issue with eating—but I still expected a forced tear or even a stern lecture. Clearly my parents had come to expect a level of drama, which included life-threatening behavior, from their only son. Either way, I was open to hearing suggestions. A parents' role is to offer guidance, unconditional love, and assist in maneuvering their closeted twelve-year-old son through anorexia, right? At last, my dad suggested that he would take the following day off from work to seek advice from a doctor.

We woke up the next morning and because my dad rarely ever had time off of work, he decided to make the most of it by suggesting that we start the day off with a father-son breakfast at my favorite greasy spoon. I was so thrilled at the thought of food that my anorexic lifestyle vanished faster than Valerie Bertinelli's career in the 90s.

I was sitting on the edge of a cold, sterile examining bed that was covered in butcher paper. I despise being naked in front of other men, then and now, for fear of the unplanned erection or drooling uncontrollably. You can imagine how comfortable I felt sitting in a see-through gown in front of my dad and a random emergency care doctor, who was so good looking he really belonged on the set of *General Hospital.*

As instructed, I lay back and held my breath as the soap opera hunk began massaging my stomach. I closed my eyes and began visualizing my grandma in order to combat the unwanted tingle I felt in my pelvic region. The doctor continued to examine my abdomen and then a rumbling of epic proportions announced itself to the room.

Doc Hollywood turned to my dad and said, "Your son is severely backed up."

"No shit, what on earth could have given you that impression?" is what I thought in my head.

"Is there something you can do for him?" My dad asked matter of fact.

"Well, have you tried a suppository?" the doctor asked, turning his head toward me.

"I don't know what that is."

My dad groaned and said, "You'll have to stick something up your butt."

"I'm okay with that if it will make me feel better." Off the reaction of my dad, I think my reply might have been too eager.

"Then it's settled," the doctor said as he pulled out his prescription pad.

After he scribbled the order and handed the prescription to my father, he began giving me a visual tutorial on how I would go about shoving the suppository up my bum.

As the doctor leaned forward and began pantomiming the action of inserting the medicine, the gravity of the procedure started to freak me out. I'd never put something up my butt before, and I knew enough from the seventh grade conversations at the lunch table that I certainly didn't want to get a reputation for starting that now!

When we got home I ran straight to the bathroom and began the shameful process. A knock at the door disturbed my disgruntled digestive efforts. It was my dad. "Do you need some help?

"No dad. Thanks, I don't want you in here."

I struggled for several minutes until I found a gentle bend in my knees, took a deep breath, and relaxed to slide the shaming suppository in. Not exactly how Dr. McHandsome demonstrated, but his visual definitely gave me something to revisit at a later time—once I was free from pain.

I sat on the toilet for well over an hour waiting for some magic movement. My dad would knock at the door every few minutes and ask the same question. "Anything?" He hadn't been this interested in my activity since I gave up soccer. "No," Was always my reply.

Finally my dad announced, "I'm coming in."

Reluctantly I invited him in to join the constipation countdown, where I sat on the toilet with my husky pants around my ankles (because at 4' 9", no matter how much weight you've lost, you're still a chunk). My dad sat next to me, trying to calm me down. Which would have been just as hard as convincing my sister to clean her room—the man had his job cut out for him.

He started telling me funny stories to get me laughing, knowing that once I began to stop thinking about the massive block, I would relax and let nature (enhanced by a suppository) do the work.

Within fifteen minutes I began to feel pokage. I knew it was going to hurt. My dad just kept talking while I pushed, and cried, and pushed, and screamed, and pushed, and cried some more—until two months' worth of crap was released—thus ending my personal miniseries perfect for Lifetime. "Starving and Constipated: A Closeted Boy's Cry For Help."

*   *   *

My senior year of high school was spectacular. Aside from my English class with Mr. Goff (which I loved) and my History class, my schedule was loaded with elective classes like Psychology, Spanish, Drama and Show Choir. I had a lot of free time to be social and creative. I also didn't care anymore about what my peers thought about me. I was friendly with almost everyone in my class, and at this point even the jocks had found a way to appreciate my sense of humor and gave up on the whole "faggot" name calling thing.

By the end of the school year the senior class stood on common ground: we had made it through hell together; now it was time to have fun! We completely embraced the fun. From our Senior Prom until the week of graduation our class overdosed on: In-school activities, bonfires, parties in the woods, and senior ditch day; all leading up to the Senior Banquet. The banquet was like the Golden Globes of high school. Everyone gathered at the "fanciest" motel pretending to be a hotel in our town, wearing their finest outfits, ready for an evening of food, dancing, awards and laughter.

I arrived that evening with a group of friends whom I had bonded with over the two years I attended Florence High School. If you saw us out together, you might question our connection; we each had a unique style, personality, and attitude—less like a clique and more like a posse. As we entered the dated lobby of the two-story motor lodge, the smell of chlorine from the indoor pool and cheap cologne from Wal-Mart overwhelmed me with excitement. It was the first time I had seen some of my Colorado classmates in something other than knockoff Northface gear and sweatpants.

The night started with the standard speeches from the adults and overachieving students who felt the need to be heard. Once we had digested our share of "inspirational" wisdom, the first course was served. Snacking on soggy salads and day old dinner rolls the energy and exchanges in the room progressed. People whom I had never talked to found their way to my table to take a minute to share a funny story or tell me that they admired my confidence. It's bizarre when the people we thought most despised us confide that they were actually jealous of us.

As we took our last bites of tasty tiramisu, the DJ cranked up the music and we rushed the dance floor. In every direction my classmates were smiling as their fists pumped in the air to Green Day. I was feeling sentimental and proud of this group of people whom I had got to know in such a short time.

The night was winding down and kids trickled out of the party. Even though I had my entire life after high school mapped out, I recognized that I was going to miss these people and this time in my life. I was desperate to keep the party going, and I started rallying people to head over to duck park (which was not the actual name of the park, but no one knew the name because the sign was covered in duck dung that had been flung by bored teenagers) to continue the high school hijinks that had bonded us in the past three hours.

My friend Amber pulled the car up to the edge of the pond where others had already started to gather, and we jumped out to join in on the fun. Without the assistance of alcohol or drugs we began running around the park as if we were celebrating Mardi Gras in the French Quarter. The park, which ran alongside the Arkansas River, was an ideal backdrop for ghost stories, hide & seek, and sexual experimentation for those "normal" seniors who weren't too busy covering up their gay urges. Basically everyone except for me and a few of my girlfriends who were smart enough to avoid unwanted teen pregnancy.

I'd spent a lot of time in class learning and laughing alongside my peers, but this evening a more meaningful relationship was formed. I was aware that we probably wouldn't stay connected—this was long before social websites, and cell phones were only used for emergencies—so unless we were going to send letters, this was our last hooray.

After a giant love-fest, the mood was starting to get somber, so I suggested that we head over to the swing-set for a friendly competition. Who could get higher and jump further? We each mounted the black plastic belt and within a few seconds the sense memory of pumping our legs transported us back to kindergarten. The mountain air was intoxicating and helped liberate us from the demands of high school's midnight cramming, pointless group projects, and exams.

Our legs vigorously pushed forward through the air as our bodies pulled back in counterbalance, up, up, up, and away. The entire swing-set started to jump and squeak from the strain of momentum. It was time to jump and (like everything I do in life), I wanted to be the first to fly free into the Universe.

I readjusted my hands into a twisted, awkward position that would help me maneuver faster. As my swing reached the apex, I engaged my core and prepped my legs for launch. "Here goes nothing!" I screamed as I released my grip of the chains and soared through the air.

Mid-air I sneezed and simultaneously farted.

Laughter from the swings erupted before my feet even touched the ground. They'd all heard the fart, but did they suspect anything else? I looked back and flipped my crew off. "I have to take a piss!" With that, I ran to the restroom.

Once safely inside the third-world facility, I frantically locked the door and took a deep breath: I had shat my pants. The only thing I could do now was clean up quickly and return to my friends. A hurricane of panic hit me when I looked down to realize there was no toilet paper—or paper towels. Thankfully, the Boy Scouts of America had taught me two things: It's okay to hook up with other boys as long as they're in uniform; and to Be Prepared. The only problem—you cannot really prepare for adult diarrhea.

My survival mode kicked into full gear. I took my pants off, pulled down my tainted underwear, and threw them in the sink. Next priority: clean my butt. I turned on the faucet, backed my backside up to the sink, and held my hand like a cup to catch the ice-cold water. I began splashing fistfuls onto my soiled bum, watching the fudge tinted runoff carefully until it was clear. Once I felt pure again, I took my underwear and attempted to wash them out. Like convincing a Republican that Liberals can care about America and still challenge leadership, I realized I was fighting an uphill battle. I discarded the mushy bottoms into the toilet—because there wasn't a trashcan—and I prayed they would flush.

Once my derriere had air-dried and my Calvin Kleins had sledged their way through the pipes, I carefully put my pants back on and exited the bathroom.

The sun was rising as I made my way back to my group of friends waiting impatiently by Amber's car.

"Where have you been?"

"Oh, I took a walk along the river. I was starting to get sad and I needed a minute by myself to take in my last night of high school."

With that outlandish lie, we all got into Amber's car to go home. When the last door was slammed shut, Amber took a deep breath and gagged, "It smells like shit in here!" Without missing a beat, I turned my head around to the back seat and said, "Which one of you assholes stepped in dog shit?!"

Traveling: New York City

When I was seventeen years old I bullied my parents into allowing me to fly to New York City to attend a pricey, but-how-can-you-not-invest-in-my-future, theater camp. At this point, my parents were living in separate states; originally for "work" my mom took a detour via Oregon while my dad, sister, and I relocated to Colorado. Eight months into the *arrangement* their impending divorce was evident yet unspoken. I needed an escape from my family, from school, from the endless self-inflicted gay shaming, and from my acne—the east coast humidity would be good for my skin.

Once again, they appeased my longwinded argument with a roundtrip ticket to musical freedom. As I boarded the airplane, I could taste the savory pizza and smell the aroma of woodsy cologne poorly masking the alcohol and cigarettes lingering on the Broadway performers from the evening before.

Five hours later, I was greeted at LaGuardia Airport by a camp volunteer who was holding a large sign with my name, accompanied by several other campers who had already arrived. After brief introductions, we loaded into a passenger van and headed to our home for the next two weeks.

I fell in love with New York the instant our van sped away from the airport and familiar landmarks materialized in every direction. We passed Shea Stadium and then suddenly I could see the New York City skyline. I knew that I was born for Broadway and now I was only

51

a car ride away. Suddenly, my dreams became blurry and so did the skyscrapers. "Why are we headed in the opposite direction of those buildings?" I blurted aloud in an alarmed and dramatic tone.

Our counselor explained that our camp was on the grounds of a university that was on Long Island and that we'd be driving into the city a handful of times to get the "full NYC experience." My hormone-filled head was spinning out of control. I couldn't understand how I'd managed to miss this towering tidbit in the brochure. Looking back I can see how a musical theater camp on Long Island seemed a lot less glamorous than one in New York City. I can understand why they neglected to highlight Hofstra's campus, choosing instead snapshots of the excursions in the city.

Strike one: I'm stuck on Long Island—along with countless other closeted theater queens.

We arrived at Hofstra University just as members of the New York Jets were making their exit from summer training camp—just like an underpaid desk clerk at a 3 Star hotel chain in Cleveland—our director asked us to wait patiently in the courtyard while our rooms were being prepared.

Strike 2: They did not offer us a cocktail while we waited. Yes, we were too young to drink, but I'd seen *Fame*, I knew that theater kids were an exception to the rules.

I made my way around the common area eager to meet as many future stars as possible. Realizing you had to act fast if you wanted to run in the hip Hofstra circle, I instantly latched onto my crew for the next two weeks. Loud, hilarious, talented, and gorgeous—would accurately describe almost every teenager who attended. I found a group that also had street smarts, wisdom (they were mostly older than I), and an outside connection to New York City.

By the time I unpacked my dorm room and swapped résumés with my new roommate, Jeromy (I'd been in more commercials, but he had more regional theater experience), it was time for our formal meet and greet. Two hundred bratty, bossy, drama geeks gathered in the main rehearsal room at Hofstra University for orientation. Once the Fear Fuhrer (AKA our camp founder) was finished lecturing us on safety, underage drinking, promiscuity, and leaving the campus without permission—which was completely verboten (and grounds for removal)—the fun began.

We mingled as if we were at the Vanity Fair Oscar party; trading celebrity gossip, boasting about our industry connections, and revealing the roles that we auditioned for but inevitably lost out to a soon-to-be-forgotten-child-star. The highlight of the evening was an informal performance featuring artists that were returning for a second season of camp. They had the entire school year to prepare bewitching monologues, dance routines, and stunning Broadway vocal solos. I thought to myself, I may be in over my head. Thankfully, my ego assured me that I would be just as remarkable at the end of the two-week intensive.

DAY 1: PLACEMENT

Just like in my favorite movie (at the time) *A Chorus Line*, we gathered in the large dance studio and learned a series of short challenging dance combinations. One at a time we performed the choreography and then advanced to the vocal placement. Because they had to process so many performers in a short amount of time, we stood in a line, and one at a time we were called to the center of the room where the musical director vocalized us at the piano. "If you can't sing scales with the piano, you probably can't sing," he declared. Thankfully, I'd been in choir since first grade and had no problem belting out the notes as he plunked away at the keys.

The moment arrived when we had to prove that we could act. One at a time the camp director had us come forward and share a funny story—real or imagined—while responding to random questions that she would challenge us with. It was a rapid-fire way of distinguishing the true professional liars (like myself) from the amateurs who struggled to remember their name.

The entire process was over in two hours, which led us right into our lunch hour. We were told that our placement would be posted in the common area following our break and that we would go directly into classes in the afternoon. I was so excited that I hardly touched my lunch, which was very out of character for me, but a happy weight loss opportunity nonetheless. The table was a buzz about the audition. We overanalyzed our performances (as dancers often do), we offered sincere praise and validation to one another (as dancers rarely do), and we contemplated our fate (as dancers always do).

Would we end up in the classes we preferred with the cool kids already in the biz? Or would we be forced to endure two weeks with the kids who would no doubt end up in the technical theater department when they discovered their creative strengths were more suited for behind the scenes duties? The stress was starting to build and carbs were my only available comfort. I dunked my Sbarro's pizza into the saucer of ranch dressing that I swiped from the salad bar, folded the slice in half, and shoved it into my mouth—just like that, my diet was over.

News of the final casting assignments spread and within minutes performers exited Hofstra's food court faster than audiences walked out of the movie *Showgirls*.

Thanks to my (then) pushy personality, I fought my way into the center of the crowd. My eyes scanned the list and I quickly located my name. "Yes! I made the "A" team," I thought in my head. Now, what about my friends? I went back to the top of the alphabetical list and discovered that Carrie L., Jenn M. and Jeromy S. were all on my list. The Four Musketeers—let the drama begin.

Carrie was a thin, beautiful Asian girl, who was as sassy as she was opinionated about everything. When she spoke, a husky no-nonsense voice dominated the conversation. She was the clear leader of our group. We called her Margret Cho, which was incredibly racist but it never dawned on us. Luckily, Carrie took this as an enormous compliment. Margret was hilarious then and continues to shine as an artist—neither her nor Carrie was afraid to confront stereotypes.

Jenn was a thin, beautiful New Yorker with a soft voice and a sparkling laugh. Her agreeable disposition offered a harmonious balance to our group. She was not a pushover and always shared her thoughts, yet she understood how to roll with the punches and made sure to enjoy every adventure along the way. She was a Zen master two years before anyone else knew the difference between sushi and feng shui.

Our final Musketeer was Jeromy, a tall, thin, oddly handsome Oklahoma City charmer. With the girls, Jeromy was flirty, cocky and ready to make out with each of them. With me, Jeromy was vying for alpha male at camp. We were both natural leaders with a competitive edge; too bad for Jeromy, my personality won over the girls faster than his swagger. In the end, the only person who really wanted to make out with Jeromy was me.

Instead, I made out with a girl who looked like Jennifer Aniston, as if I were on the set of the breakout television hit of the year, *Friends*. Even though I wore sweater-vests (regularly) I did not identify with

Chandler and his lack of charm. *Joey* was super hot, which was a perk, but he was entirely too stupid for me to latch onto. Which left me with neurotic, whining, Ross—whom I completely understood—and hence made perfect sense for me to pretend date *Rachel*… at theater camp [Beat] on Long Island.

DAY 3: FINDING OUR GROOVE

At this point everyone was comfortably situated in their dance, music, and acting classes. The Four Musketeers dominated our rehearsals during the day and mastered the social scene at night. The camp counselors went out of their way to keep us entertained with VHS tapes of over-watched 80's films, boring board games, and tame treasure hunts, but the true adventures came after "lights out." There in the darkness of the dank dorm rooms we gathered in a circle playing rounds of Truth or Dare and Spin the Bottle. There was a lot of girl on girl action due to the low boy to girl ratio, I kept praying that my bottle would land on Jeromy to even out the score, and instead I got stuck making out with one of the more desperate ingénues at camp. She was cute enough and the kiss was all right, but I still had to close my eyes and think about Paul Rudd a la *Clueless*. It was only my second French kiss; my first was at Tina Falconie's eight grade graduation party. There in the clubhouse in Tina's backyard I was sent to Seven Minutes in Heaven with an adorably shy and intelligent girl named Heather. I'll never forget Heather's reaction when my tongue passed through her sweet, soft, innocent lips. "Gross, what are you doing?" "I'm kissing you. This is how you do it…" I replied, terrified that as a closeted gay boy I couldn't even get that right.

"Why don't you just braid my hair instead?"

"Okay, but can I at least feel your boobs first?" It's been my experience that all men—gay or straight—have a mad infatuation with fleshy bouncing breasts. I'm not trying to be insensitive or sexualize women, I'm positive it's an instinctual reaction.

DAY FIVE: OFF CAMPUS—PASS

At the end of the first week we owned our environment. The fantastic four were clearly untouchable amongst the other thespians. We excelled in the lead roles and hosted the best late night soirées— the fame was going to our heads.

Carrie was starting to get antsy and decided to raise the bar by suggesting that we sneak out to the 24 hour Dunkin' Donut/Chinese restaurant hybrid. Jeromy was quick to say yes. But Jenn and I had some trepidation. I was always on board for a wild adventure, but I'd spent my entire life taking calculated risks.

For example, I might lead a team of teenagers to toilet paper a frienemy's house, but I'd make sure to plan the attack on a weekend I was sure the family was out of town. Or I'd rally my entire Boy Scout pack to sneak from the boys' side of the overnight beach camp to the girls' side, where the Southern California chapter of the Girl Scouts of America awaited our midnight mayhem. However, I was prepared with a roll of toilet paper and a flashlight, so that when our scout leaders caught us I could sneak away from the rest of the pack and pretend that I was just strolling back from a late night bowel break. I had a mild obsession with T. P. as a teenager.

After a long pause, I decided to throw caution to the wind and join my musical mates for a jaunt in Long Island. It was easy slipping out of the dorm room and past the campus security guard, who was busy taking a catnap. Once we were off campus, we crossed the motionless street and made our way over to the combination chain restaurant. Aside from the homeless man who sat just outside the front door, the place was empty. I studied the menu carefully, making sure to spend my money on the precise combination of salty and sweet that I craved at 2 a.m. I was the last to order and as I walked up to the counter I heard Carrie instruct us, "Just stay calm." What was she talking about? As I began to order my Beef and Broccoli and two maple-glazed Long Johns (one for dessert and the other for breakfast), I saw two police officers out of the corner of my eye. My balls retracted into my skull and my heart replaced their presence in my ball sack. I casually paid the cashier my money, passed the police officers flashing a huge smile, and walked over to join Carrie, Jen, and Jeromy who were now talking about their faux term papers for History class. Reminder: It was the middle of summer.

The officers returned the smile as they walked to the counter and ordered two black coffees. Would they take us straight to the police station? Or would they walk us back to the campus and wake up our dorm room counselors? I was running through a list of lies I might tell the officers if confronted: "We suffer from group sleepwalking disorder or GSD." Or "We couldn't take the heavy demands of theater camp, so our parents told us to meet them here to defect." More believable still: "They aren't feeding us enough food during the day and our bodies *needed* the extra sustenance."

To our good fate, New York's finest (and they were hot in a Chippendales way) grabbed their coffees and headed toward the door. The taller and hotter of the two turned back before exiting and said, "You kids be safe out there tonight."

We exhaled in unison, grabbed our bag of greasy goodness and headed back to Hofstra. In the wee hours of the morning I woke up to a revolutionary discovery that I would carry with me for the rest of my life: when you smile, keep your cool, and act like you belong—no body questions you.

We hadn't devised a plan to sneak back onto campus, so we were utterly caught off guard when we heard the campus security guard's husky voice say, "Just where do you think you're going?" Confidently I offered, "Hey, we just stepped out for a late night snack. It's cool, we cleared it with our dorm monitor before leaving."

"There are no off campus privileges for summer camps students; NO exceptions."

Now feeling very brave (because we had nothing to lose at this point) I said, "Well, we managed to get off campus without your knowledge—perhaps because you were sleeping on the job—so technically our problem is also YOUR problem. But nobody has to know if we keep this between us. Plus, I have an extra Long John that I'm happy to share with you; think of it as a hall pass."

Officer Mayberry accepted the sticky bribe in exchange for his silence—another life lesson learned.

Safely in our dorm room we inhaled our Chinese food and agreed that it tasted better than any we'd had before. Was it because we narrowly escaped prison or just extra MSG? Like the restaurant from which it came, I think it was a combination.

DAY 7: SHIT POOPIE

I was lying on my back in a cold black box theater listening to Liza Genero ramble on about inviting light in to my body through my hands and feet while thinking my parents paid a lot of money for this nonsense. I came to theater camp to sing and dance, not learn about spirituality from a Broadway legend's daughter…Twenty minutes into class she finally had us up on our feet learning box steps. I mean seriously, a box step? My dad could do a box step in his sleep, while changing a toilet and calking at the bathroom sink. This was outrageous!

"Make sure you know this choreography inside and out, because in a moment we're going to add the lyrics and it's really going to throw you off!" she said, trying to assure herself that this was a challenge for anyone over the age of two.

She handed us the sheet music to start learning the lyrics. Our group had been assigned "Shipoopi" from the musical *The Music Man*. We gathered around the piano and even faster than we picked up the box step, we collectively learned the three verses and repeating chorus in about five minutes. Like a first-time mother trying to motivate her child to eat peas, she excitedly clapped her hands together and said, "Okay, let's try to put this all together."

I looked over at Carrie and rolled my eyes. Carrie responded with a snarky smile and pantomimed an exuberant clap with her hands. We danced and sang our bored faces off. When we got to the third chorus I was ready for a little light-hearted humor to cheer up the room. Rather than singing the written lyrics, I added a "T" to the end of every "shi" of shipoopi (not a creative or far reaching stretch for a smart ass teenager) and belted out "Sssshit-poopi, SHIT-poopi, the girl who's hard to get. Ssssshit-poopi, SHIT-poopi, but you can win her yet." Suddenly there was an outburst of laughter and everyone butchered the box step.

Liza walked over to me, stood directly in front of me, and (similar to the day before, when she asked me stand in front of my peers and sing my solo, while berating my technique) screamed at me and told me that I was, "Never going to make it as a performer because I lacked discipline."

I took a deep breath and looked her in the eyes. Even then, I could see that she was projecting her insecurities onto me. I smiled and said, "Well, that's your opinion. Not that it matters much, you're teaching kids at a summer camp instead of choreographing an *actual* Broadway show." I took no issue with a theater professional yielding their career from the cutthroat competition of the legitimate stage to share their wisdom and passion as an educator, so long as they do so with some integrity.

She kicked me out of the class, but not before I could say, "Good! Because this choreography is SHIT! [Beat] poopi!"

DAY 8: BROADWAY BOUND

After apologizing to Liza in a one-on-one meeting in the camp director's office, I was allowed to rejoin the not-even-remarkable-enough-to-choreograph-community-theater choreographer and the rest of my cast to continue rehearsing her piece. At least I'd get to perform with my friends in the showcase. Camp was nearing an end, which meant we (FINALLY) got to go into the city for a Broadway show, sightseeing and dinner.

Comfortably seated on the big yellow bus and heading toward the skyline my parents paid top dollar for me to enjoy, one of the counselors stood up and announced the show we'd be attending was *How To Succeed In Business Without Really Trying* starring Matthew Broderick and a then-lesser-known Megan Mullally (please see *Faced With Fame* to read about my full circle moment with the vivacious Karen Walker).

The smell of ambition and male construction worker sweat in the summer humidity greeted us in Manhattan and we were early enough to enjoy some window-shopping and check out a few dance classes at Broadway Dance Center before our matinee at the Richard Rodgers Theatre.

Taking our seats on the orchestra level, I studied my Playbill the same way I watched my dad examine baseball players batting averages in the Scorecard at Dodger's Stadium. Line by line I combed every biography, cross-referencing credits and scrutinizing head shots—I could rank the performers and their talent prior to seeing them on stage, based on their bio and picture alone. Before the show even began, the theater was alive with the harmonious sound of drama geeks gushing over their favorite Broadway performers. Then, the lights went down and the orchestra swelled.

We heard *Ferris Bueller's* voice before we saw Matthew Broderick ascend from the fly space at the top of the proscenium of the stage. My adrenalin was pumping as Matthew was slowly lowered on a platform like a window washer outside a high-rise office building. I was instantly baited into the story of a young man's aspirations and calculated advancement from a window washer to chairman of the board in corporate America. The story was relatable and mirrored my own internal feelings. Why climb the corporate ladder if you already have access to the executive suite? The music and lyrics were both catchy and clever in developing the plot. The choreography was grounded, stylized, and complimented the story with a vibrant energy. The entire cast of triple threats shone, including a stand out performance from Megan Mullally, who played Broderick's love interest.

Directly after the performance we were surprised with a private meet and greet with the cast. We were told that Matthew would not be able to join us. Regardless, several members of the ensemble, Megan, and Lillias White (also a Broadway legend who sang her face off) met us in the house after their performance to share advice and answer annoying teenage questions like: "What's it like to work with Matthew Broderick?" "Do any of you *get* to hang out with Matthew Broderick?" And "Does Matthew Broderick ever talk about *Ferris Bueller's Day Off*?"

In hindsight I can see how irked these talented professionals must have been. They'd just finished a dazzling performance and instead of taking a break to rest between shows, they went out of their way to come out and talk to a bunch of teenaged musical theater hopefuls. Rather than using our time to ask practical questions about training, auditions, or the life of a Broadway performer, we focused on the one star who hadn't joined the discussion.

Suddenly from the stage right wing we saw Matthew. He walked out and took center stage in the middle of a response from Lillias, and in the same way that Oprah's audience used to react to her annual "Favorite Things" show, we lost our shit.

Matthew and his winning grin welcomed a few questions before—in true Ferris fashion—the stage manager stepped onto the stage with an "urgent message" for Mr. Broderick. Taking their cue from Matthew's exit, the entire cast exited the scene to prepare for their evening performance.

Enjoying a full-body high from the tremendous show and follow up Q&A, I levitated down the street and over to the Hard Rock Café with my gang of musical theater gurus. Consuming French fries, burgers, and coffee milkshakes at the overpriced but in vogue themed restaurant, our crew took turns sharing their favorite highlights from the performance. Most of my friends (who were from the New York area) spoke as if they were ordained theater critics. I unapologetically gushed over the performances, swooned about the music, and raved about my favorite part—the choreography. "I thought Wayne Cilento did a magnificent job capturing the feeling of the music and lyrics." Met with a table full of eye rolls, I learned a third life lesson: theater people were hilarious, creative, loud, obnoxious, and unable to appreciate someone else's work until ten other critics do so in print.

DAY 10: BYE BYE BROADWAY

The energy on the morning of our final day of camp was schizophrenic. Enthusiastic to share our performances during the showcase and at the same time the somber awareness that we would be saying goodbye to our newfound comrades was *Les Misérables!*

I finished packing my trunk the night before so that I could spend as much time with Carrie, Jen, and Jeromy as possible, laughing and rehearsing for our big debut. Over lunch we conspired to stay in touch with one another—Jeromy and I both had one more year of school left—before we could move to New York City and share an apartment with one another. Carrie and Jen were both headed to New York University. It was two years before email addresses were readily accessible (and long before social media) so instead we swapped addresses and phone numbers with every intention of remaining lifelong musical mates.

Sadly, by the end of our showcase performance (where I sang "shit-poopi" under my breath at least three times just because I could), Jeromy was already over our friendship when I was awarded the Male Performer Most Likely to Appear on Broadway. I guess some people can't handle the truth—even in a mock circumstance.

I hugged Carrie and Jen for at least ten minutes before being ripped away by an angry counselor whose patience for our personalities had run out on the second day of camp. I cried for the entire bus ride to the airport, and then stepping onto the airplane I adopted a more mature, confident posture and attitude.

After flying across the country by myself, meeting like-minded people, narrowly escaping jail time, indulging in MSG, enduring a diva choreographer who hated my spirit, gaining inspiration from Broadway performers, and receiving praise for my performance at a camp that grooms performers—I no longer felt anxiety about the problems I was dealing with back home. Suddenly it became clear that I was in control of my own life. Rather than running away from my fears, I would unabashedly sing and dance my way towards them. It was my first "I don't give a fuck" moment, and instantly I decided that this would be my mantra for the rest of my life.

P.S. Jen and I exchanged one letter after camp and then lost touch. Carrie and I spent four months corresponding until the demands of her classes at NYU proved too time consuming. I've searched for both of them on Facebook and cannot find either of them; Jeromy on the other hand, is on the social media website and though we share mutual connections—we are not friends.

Traveling: Texas

I was six years old and in search of the perfect Father's Day gift for my dad. The florescent bulbs and wire racks in the novelty shops that littered Main Street—before megastores destroyed local economies—exposed T-shirts, key chains, BBQ aprons, and coffee mugs declaring: "The World's Greatest Dad." Predictable plastic praise from an average son to his father, but I was not *average,* and my dad *is* the world's greatest dad. Even then I knew that the low quality merchandise in these stores was unsuitable for my hero.

I wanted to join Cub Scouts when I was eight. My dad, Tony, became the Den Leader and celebrated my boyhood right of passage by purchasing me a red Swiss Army Knife. *MacGyver* was a popular television show at the time. Richard Dean Anderson, the star of the show, was so hot—and handy with a knife—and I now owned my very own mini weapon. The weight and functionality of the Swiss-made cutlery felt heavy in my palm; naturally I wanted to show off. I brought my handy tool to school and when my third grade teacher caught me deactivating a faux explosive device behind the gym, my dad had to come and bail me out. With his back turned away from Mrs. Oberwater as he reprimanded me, I caught the sparkle in his eyes: he was proud.

When I would feign sickness to avoid a test or a bully at school he would come home from work with Snickers bars and video game magazines to lift my spirits. I was eight when I watched Halley's Comet pass in the night sky with my dad by my side.

He was my lab assistant for every Science Fair Project from third through eighth grade, proving—among many things—that Science was not my strong suit, plants *do* need sunlight to survive, and when working on projects that involve balsa wood or flammable chemicals you should expect spontaneous explosions between fathers and sons.

I started a coin collection in the sixth grade and he encouraged my hobby by investing in a hefty coin guide. When I decided to paint several of the precious coins with finger nail polish, adding a pop of color to my collection, he complimented the vibrant choice.

In eighth grade I climbed to the top of a towering water park slide in an attempt to impress my buddies. When I reached the peak of the colossal waterway and panicked, he paid me $20 to brave the freefall, rather than facing defeat by descending back down the stairs.

Secretly jealous of the shin guards that caressed the muscular legs of my peers, I decided to play soccer. My dad signed up as the coach and led our team to regional victory. When I bailed on soccer in order to take dance classes instead, he gave me two thumbs up. And when, as a freshman, I enrolled myself and was accepted into a performing arts high school (thirty miles from our house) he smiled and drove me to and from school every day, adding an extra hour to his work day.

No surprise, then, that when I reached the end of my senior year and begged to skip three days of school to attend an audition in Dallas, Texas—my dad cashed in his vacation days from work, signed the attendance release form, and gassed up the Jeep. Road trip!

My dad—a plumbing contractor—is a man's man with traditional Christian values. I'm sure this was not exactly the road trip that he had envisioned sharing with his only son, who would soon be leaving home. Perhaps driving cross country for: a deep sea fishing expedition, a football training camp, rock climbing in the Grand Canyon, or downhill mountain biking in Moab (which we actually did the following month) would have been more appealing. To his credit, my dad pulled out the map and plotted our course from Florence, Colorado to Dallas, Texas. Like a good Boy Scout, he was always prepared to fulfill his fatherly duties.

The next evening, when my dad got home from work, I piled into the passenger seat of our well-worn Jeep Cherokee. Two of my fellow dance mates, Maria and Jennifer—who were also desperate to book work as a performer upon graduation—piled into the back of our SUV, and we headed toward Texas. Dad decided to drive the nightshift, which was the larger, scarier part of the journey, and we would split the remaining daylight portion of our voyage into the Deep South.

The terrain in the United States can be majestic. Mountains covered in varying shades of green that contrast huge grey boulders balancing on the tiniest ledges. Deserts surrounded by shelves of multicolored red, pink, and orange rock with oddly shaped cacti and whimsical trees that look like they're straight out of a Dr. Seuss book. Rolling fields of yellow that catch the wind convincing you that the ocean is made of grain. This stretch of America was none of that.

The road was straighter than Tom Selleck and the land as flat as every joke a politician delivers during an election season to enhance their likeability. The *Inconvenient Truth* is that not even Al Gore could inspire people to travel through this part of our country, and my dad was forced to because his closeted-gay son (and his besties) *needed* to get to an audition and didn't have enough money for a last minute airplane ticket.

In order to make the long desolate drive more enjoyable my dad cranked *Eagles* cassette tapes, which he had stockpiled in the center console, and the four of us belted high notes at the top of our lungs. Who knew the *Eagles* would spark such an unlikely musical bond between generations? My dad, that's who. The music was an interactive way to pass time, but more so, the beautiful melodies and expressive lyrics appealed to our artistic spirits.

Although he might not acknowledge it today, my dad was an artist himself. He played the trumpet through school, and even now, he'll sit down at the piano and play while singing (mostly) off key, but always out loud and proud.

Born in the late 50s, his childhood was shaped by images of John F. Kennedy, Martin Luther King, Nixon, Mao, Che, the Civil Rights Movement, Vietnam, and Neil Armstrong becoming the first human to walk on the moon. It played out before his eyes with a soundtrack from the likes of Bob Dylan, *The Beach Boys*, *Simon and Garfunkel*, *The Rolling Stones*, Johnny Cash, *The Who*, *Fleetwood Mac*, and of course *The Beatles*. By the time he had reached his formative teenage years, he was a free-loving, thrill seeking, outdoor hippie dude of the 70s with a new sound; the *Eagles*.

Somewhere on highway 87 during the song *Hotel California*, I learned that my dad had a girlfriend before my mom—or my aunt.

A long-standing family joke, that my dad took my mom's sister to his senior prom before my parents became a couple. Even before that though, my dad was head over heels about another girl. He claimed it never got serious because she had a lot of emotional problems—my dad has always had a soft spot for a damsel in distress.

"I can't recall. I'm sure I met your mom [who was two years his junior] and she swept me off my feet." This was his only response when I grilled him for more details about his first love.

Sadly, his first girlfriend passed away from a drug overdose years after they'd graduated high school, so I guess he dodged a bullet there. Also, I might never have been born. Still, I could sense my dad's discontent. Not because he ended up with my mom, but because he had failed himself by not rescuing a broken spirit. He would save his worst enemy if ever put in that position.

When my family uprooted from California to Colorado my junior year, Maria became my first new friend. Not that it was ever hard for me to make friends, but at this point in my life, I *knew* that I was going to be a professional dancer. Maria was the only other high school student who seemed to have her life figured out. We were comrades in dance. Maria was a quiet, sensitive soul but her petite frame packed a mean punch. As prone to laughter as she was to a sudden outburst of moodiness, she was layered and complicated—just like an artist should be. She was an expressive dancer, with big brown eyes that tried to hide behind her jet black long blunt bangs. Her lines were shockingly elegant, but it was the intensity behind her attack that left audiences in awe when she performed.

Like a true dancer, Maria spoke with her body language more than her mouth. Not even her closest friends could convince her that she was in a safe space to talk freely. Did I mention she was a very wise person? It was during our tenth hour on the road that Maria conveyed her fear of being stuck in a small town for the rest of her life with no hope of traveling the world and performing; the only thing that she truly desired.

Jennifer on the other hand was an open book full of opinions and never bashful about expressing them. She was a tall, blonde ballerina with a natural facility and effortless talent. Born into an affluent family in Southern Colorado, she had access to any path that she desired in life. She was confident, sharp, and bitingly funny. If anyone was born to be a dancer, it was Jennifer, which is why it left us astonished when she confessed that she'd sooner get married and have babies with her boyfriend than pursue a professional career.

Whether it was the *Eagles*, the bleak scenery, or the preservatives from the gas station snacks we consumed, my eyes were opened in a way they hadn't been before. Between every service station and rest stop the four of us would take turns sharing our fears, dreams, and regrets. (I'm still furious that I traded my entire Garbage Pail Kids card collection for two Grandma's Homestyle fudge chocolate chip cookies and a King Size bag of Funyuns, in the fourth grade.) This expedition became my transition into adulthood. I started to process how complicated the human psyche is. It was the first time I accepted my father as a human—with thoughts, dreams, and fears of his own—and not just my "dad".

Full of junk food and a newfound respect for one another, we rolled into Dallas with just enough time to check in at the motel, take a shower, and get dressed in our audition wardrobe. After getting lost (three times) my dad finally pulled into the parking lot of the University of Texas, Dallas.

My stomach was rumbling from pre-audition nerves as we jumped out of the car and ran toward the theater entrance. The casting announcement placed in the Metro section of the Denver Post the week prior was very unclear about what to expect. Aside from a date, time, and location, we had very little information other than: "Seeking high energy dancers proficient in ballet and jazz. Singing is a plus, but not a requirement. ALL DANCERS must be 18 years of age and will be required to wear costumes with limited vision."

I was the first to arrive in the lobby of the theater, where an unfriendly assistant explained that there was only ten minutes to spare before the male dancers were called in. I printed my name on the audition sign-in log, handed over my picture and résumé, and filled out an extensive size sheet.

Maria and Jennifer had a few hours to spare, but decided to sit in the back of the theater with my dad to watch the process.

I walked onto the enormous stage, which looked even larger because there were only four other guys auditioning, and we waited. Near the stage right wing there was a weathered black grand piano with a funny gentleman at the helm. We made small talk with Rob, who was later introduced as the musical director, until finally the director (who was also the choreographer) approached us.

She was a no-nonsense New York diva. Her legs said Fosse, but her face said Hitler. She introduced herself as Linda, gave us a brief synopsis of the show, and concluded with, "just have fun, show me your personality, and don't fuck up the steps."

Linda formally introduced us to Rob, who handed us lyrics for the opening number. She made it very clear that we should learn the melody and lyrics quickly, because we would be adding complicated choreography soon after.

Rob plunked out the melody note by note, emphasizing each lyric. Without question, he knew his way around a "dancer-singer". He was specific in which lyrics should be sustained or staccato, based on the choreography and our ability to remain on pitch. After several rounds of *We Need A Little Christmas,* it was obvious that two of the men *needed* a little voice lesson—thankfully, I was not one of them—because our last time through the song, we each had to sing it solo.

Once Linda had "heard enough" she jumped into teaching the choreography. The dated 80s jazz was more awkward than it was *challenging*. Good news for me, I'd spent enough summers at theater camps digesting the thoughtless work of many a jaded choreographer before her, to understand that my only job was to make her clumsy choreographic work look good.

She taught the combination fairly quickly, and then spent another forty minutes re-teaching the phrase for the two men who must have considered themselves stronger *actors* than dancer-singers.

Finally it was time to perform. Beyond the beaming heat of the stage lights, I could see my dad, Maria, and Jennifer rooting for me at the back of the theater. My dad looked nervous as he shifted in his seat, which only added to my jitters.

There were only five of us auditioning, so Linda decided that we would each do the combination one at a time. I'm not exaggerating when I tell you that I was the only performer who finished the combination. One of the men stopped in the middle of the combination and started reciting a monologue that I'm pretty sure was from the movie *Die Hard*. Which despite auditioning for a Christmas show made sense, because that is exactly what he was doing.

After each of us had the privilege of competing one at a time, she asked three of the men to leave. I was asked to stay with another young man who was a good dancer, but had trouble remembering the choreography. We learned a more technical ballet combination in a very short amount of time, and again, she had us each perform it on our own.

The moment of truth came when Linda called us over and expressed that she "very much enjoyed our stage presence and our clean execution," elaborating that she was afraid we both looked too young to cast in a show alongside older, more *seasoned*, men.

Just like that, my dream was crushed. Through tears, I watched from the back of the theater as Maria and Jennifer danced rings around the other ladies. I knew them intimately now and I was impressed with their skill, confidence, and talent. They soared through the air, floated across the stage en pointé, and sang in the Christmas cheer; in the end they, too, met my youthful fate.

I was embarrassed and discontented that we had traveled so far and failed. Without missing a beat my dad suggested that we check out the Dallas nightlife. He quickly flipped the tone of our day and rallied us to get pumped up about a dinner at the Hard Rock Café, because which teenager in the 90s wouldn't jump at the chance to score another pin for their collection? Oh yeah, did I mention that my dad and I collected souvenir pins, too?

While eating our overpriced burgers my dad shared how impressed he was with us.

"I could never do what you guys did today. Performing in front of a big-time director while they critique you? That's a terrifying thing, and all three of you rose to the occasion."

Suddenly I felt accomplished. Not just because I had swallowed a mouthful of cheese-covered French fries dipped in Ranch dressing, but because my dad was proud of me; and he confirmed it aloud in a hokey, middle class themed restaurant.

Whether we were backpacking for two weeks through the Los Angeles Mountains, bridge jumping in the heartland of Colorado, or trekking 800 miles across the southwest for an audition, my dad has never missed a moment to build up my confidence and character. By trade, he's a blue-collar boss who left school—and surrendered his silent hope of becoming an Oceanographer—to raise a family and encourage their dreams. By example, he is a leader full of courage, integrity, and wisdom.

My dad goaded me to continue auditioning for Linda, convinced that I would eventually earn her respect and a spot in the show. Either she didn't like me, or she never saw me as anything other than the inexperienced, under seasoned boy who first auditioned for her in Texas, but she never cast me in the touring show. Fortuitous for me, four years later, I auditioned for the New York City director, and landed a coveted spot in *The Christmas Spectacular* at Radio City Music Hall.

When I looked out into the audience past the flock of holiday enthusiasts who filled the 6,000-seat theater, I could see my dad sitting Orchestra center—he was gleaming with pride. I had finally found the perfect gift for the world's greatest dad, and it wasn't something that was manufactured in China. I was honored that I could give him the present of following through and manifesting my dreams, so that his sacrifice wasn't in vain. And just for good measure, I bought him a plastic commemorative Radio City souvenir, too!

Missed
COCKortunities

I left Chicago for a four-month tour of Europe as a bright-eyed, eager, virgin dancer boy and returned a full-fledged company man. Getting touched on tour was not something that just happened to me; I encourage it. Whether it was subconscious or blatant, it felt decadent and devious. It was also long overdue. Looking back at the list of guys who were evidently eager about allowing me to explore my forbidden feelings with their body parts is staggering. Only now—in my proudly out and married life—can I acknowledge the colossal COCKortunities I missed.

* * *

I was thirteen years old when I booked a role dancing in a Japanese commercial with eleven other dancers. Together we made up a little league team, because nothing says "American Beef" (the subject of the commercial) like a room full of pre-pubescent male dancers pretending to be baseball players.

After three days of choreography and music rehearsals, the time came to shoot on the location of a minor league baseball stadium in Long Beach, California. My parents both worked fulltime jobs, thus they would go out of their way to befriend a stage mom (or dad) during the final callbacks of any project I was being considered for. This surrogate mom-ager would look after me while my mom and dad were busy earning less money than I, for the day.

Joey's mom was your average LA stage mom: outgoing, loud, and unafraid to ruffle feathers on a set. She provided the perfect watchdog eye over me, and in return, I kept an even closer eye on her hot, blond, talented son.

Joey never missed an opportunity to show off during a rehearsal break. He would find every excuse to touch as many of the boys as possible; it was clear he was pitching for my team and uninhibited about swinging his bat around.

On the day of our shoot, we were all crowded into the dugout waiting for the camera crew to set up the shot. The sexual tension was more prominent than the lingering smell of jock-sweat and chewing tobacco, which only increased our growing curiosities. Naturally, for a bunch of thirteen-year-old (most likely gay) dancers pretending to be major leaguers, our conversation turned to foul play and Joey was the team captain of raising the wood. Just around the time that we were all near a grand slam in our pants, the assistant director came over to relocate us to the men's locker room. Big mistake!

Once inside the even more erotic locker bay, we were told to change into our costumes, which had been hung (pun intended) in lockers with our corresponding names.

I quickly grabbed my costume, baseball jersey and knickers, and headed toward the private stalls on the other side of the men's locker room. I felt the uninvited presence of Joey as he quickly jumped in and shut the stall door behind us. I turned and made direct contact with his sky-blue seductive eyes, his full-red-upper lip curled up as he grinned and asked if I needed some help. My heart and groin said yes, but my knee reacted instinctually to preserve my straight game. My kneecap was in his nuts. As a thirteen-year-old I was no good at throwing balls, but I was an MVP at crushing them.

* * *

My senior year of high school I decided to become a peer councilor. I loved gossiping, telling people what to do, having my own office (shared with six other peer councilors), and I was thrilled to fill my remaining non-elective period with an "easy" A.

During my sessions that year, I discovered that: the most intelligent girl in our senior class was pregnant; no matter how popular or disliked, all teenagers are insecure about fitting in; everyone masturbates—a lot; and that Joe Rich decided that I was a *safe* person to "come out" to, because I could sympathize with his pain.

He slunk into my office with a desperate gravity similar to most of the troubled souls seeking the ear of a judgmental peer. He was kind and struggled to say the words aloud. I listened attentively, making mental notes, everything that he was saying rang true in my heart and in my pants, and yet the moment he was done sharing his truth, I looked him directly in the eye and told him that I could never understand where he was coming from.

He placed his hand firmly on my shoulder, leaned in brushing his stubble (one of the few seniors with facial hair) against the side of my peach-fuzzed cheek, and whispered in my ear, "I think you know exactly what I'm talking about." I could feel the hairs on the back of my neck stand to attention, replicating the erection in my pants.

I calmly sat down—attempting to hide the evidence against my case—and asked him to leave my office. I informed our peer supervisor, who was also the school's guidance councilor, that I would no longer be able to see Mr. Rich. I explained that we had a different set of moral guidelines—I was a good Catholic boy who would do anything to suppress my inner feelings to avoid an eternity in Hell, and Joe was the Devil. That was the end of that.

* * *

Lying on the floor of my four hundred square foot apartment the morning after a wild party, I felt his fingers come in contact with mine. I was only five months removed from living under my parents' roof, still eighteen, and on my own with a handsome hunk I'd just met through a mutual friend.

We had utterly too much to drink the night before, and Mark asked if he could crash with me at my place. Our friend, Gina, was a slob and he didn't really feel clean sleeping at her place, which was just two floors down in the same building that we appropriately named "Hellrose Place" after the popular nighttime soap opera *Melrose Place*. I didn't need an excuse to say yes. His gorgeous face, dark brown hair, six-pack abs that peeked through his skintight designer button-down, and high, tight, ample ass were all I needed.

I could feel Mark's energy throughout the night slowly inching closer to the sixty-dollar futon mattress I called a bed. Aside from the lack-luster dry humping and make-out sessions I had with my high school girlfriend, I had never actually experienced the touch of another person in an erotic way. Mark embarked on a sensual exploration that would lead to an explosion in my pants and a warning at work.

At three o' clock in the morning (I remember the time because I looked up at my VCR to torture myself with the how-many-hours-of-sleep-can-I-get-before-I-have-to-be-at-work game) I could feel Mark's leg brushing up against mine. Throughout the seedy hours of darkness he continued to challenge my personal space with casual encounters.

I lived on the top floor of the eight-story complex and my apartment had a huge industrial bay window that flooded my studio apartment with sunlight at the crack of dawn every day.

Normally the harsh direct heat was overbearing, but served as the perfect wake-up call for my morning shift as a host at the popular breakfast eatery, Le Peep. This particular morning the rays illuminated the inescapable fact that I was blowing off work for a boy.

His hands were entangled with mine and his right leg was completely wrapped around my torso—like a game of Twister—he continued to invade my body. I felt his hands exploring my lower back, rapidly approaching the elastic band of my FTL underwear. He caressed my back, buttocks, and neck for another fifteen minutes before he finally persuaded me to roll over, where he continued his handy work along my stomach and legs, but noticeably avoiding my manhood.

During the course of the entire escapade I kept my head fixed facing in the opposite direction, silently declaring that *this* physical act might be happening, but I am not acknowledging it. Finally, Mark stopped fondling my body and turned to me, "I don't get it—why haven't you kissed me yet?"

Trust me, the urge to kiss Mark was undeniable, but years of crucifying myself for having these feelings had caused a major split personality in my pants. I had only kissed a handful of girls, none of whom ever touched me the way Mark did, so I never had the desire to explore what came after second base.

I had this beautiful boy lying next to me waiting to be kissed, coupled with a burning desire to jump his body and study every chiseled muscle; instead I sprung to my feet and jumped into a cold shower. Without saying a word, I dressed and rushed off to Le Peep.

After an hour of replaying the savory saga in my head while serving rich college kids their overpriced eggs, I decided that I would apologize to Mark and attempt to explain my situation when I returned home. No sooner had I arrived at my decision, than fate intervened; Gina and Mark were walking toward the host counter.

"Whatareyoudoinghere?" IaskedGinainaguiltyanddesperatetone. Having no clue what happened the night before, Gina assured me that they were here to enjoy breakfast before Mark returned to California.

My spirit sank as I watched them laugh over French toast. I wanted to be the guy sitting across from the boy who had spent the morning making me feel loved, special, appreciated, and normal. Instead, my misinformed, sanctimonious, and fear-based self-denial prevented me from walking over to offer more coffee.

* * *

Not long after my experience with Mark another brush with bromance occurred. This time I was more prepared for the aggressive stroking, but in the end I couldn't handle the supersized equipment.

Jonathan was a scholarship student at the dance company where I had an apprenticeship. I was captivated by his self-confidence. He was not afraid to show off his personality in the form of flamboyant plaid prints and micro-booty-shorts—and his body wore everything like Mark Wahlberg rocked a pair of Calvin Kleins in the 90s.

For several weeks we would exchange sassy banter during dance classes and make playful eye contact between rehearsals, which lead to a steamy evening after one of my concerts.

Following our final Chicago performance, I could see Jonathan standing off-stage-left gazing directly at me while I stepped forward to take my final bow. I could hardly wait to get off stage and get off.

Once I had showered and changed into my best "straight-boy" outfit (I was still buying clothes that were two sizes too big) I hurried out to the lobby where all of the scholarship dancers waited for the company members. I was still a performing apprentice and not yet a full-fledged company member, which left me with a choice: do I slum it with the other scholarship dancers who I attend daily classes with or do I elevate my status alongside the company members with whom I perform? The company members, most of whom were well into their twenties and early thirties, unequivocally have more fun; they have access to alcohol. In the end, their cosmopolitan cocktails didn't measure up to Jonathan's hometown charm, so I broke rank to hangout with the hottie.

One fake ID and several cash contributions later, the scholarship students scored a bottle of Malibu Rum. We took turns chugging while twirling on a merry-go-round in a park near the theater until Jonathan offered up his apartment for an after-party.

Safe in the sanctity of Jonathan's living room we continued to discuss things that catty young dancers do. Who looked fat in their costumes? How did so-and-so get hired for another season? And who would be our celebrity fuck from the cast of *Friends?* The gossip and laughter continued for hours until people started crashing. I was too infatuated to sleep. My previous heavy petting pal, Mark, was the appetizer that no one knew about. The question before me: Was I unequivocally prepared to sample the entrée (and Jonathan was one hot dish) in an apartment full of my peers?

It started off small. We were sitting across from one another and he stretched his leg out to brush his foot against mine. I could feel the strength of his body in his pinky toe as it wrapped around the arch of my foot. He slowly crawled toward me and before I knew it, he was on top of me. I wasn't ready to kiss him yet, enthusiastically Jonathan was willing to focus on his prep work; kissing my cheek, neck, finally making his way to my torso.

Fearing that one of our friends would wake up to find us devouring each other, I suggested that we move our activity to his bedroom. I could see his eyes light up and I felt an instant panic: "Oh know, does he think I'm going to have sex with him." I'd spent nineteen years lying to myself—I. AM. NOT. GAY! Sex was not on the menu for me, but I rode my Malibu rum induced wave down the hallway and into his bedroom.

Once inside, I couldn't resist the urge I felt to take off his clothes and stare at his naked body—which is exactly what I did—STUDying his smooth, toned skin and stunning masculinity. He reached over and pulled me on top of him.

He took off my shirt but I wouldn't let him remove my pants. I had my boundaries and I refused to give in. My burdened conscience and holier-than-thou attitude had reached critical mass. My family and friends would judge me, and my life—as a famous actor—would be over before it started all because of my lust for the same sex. Not even alcohol freed me to kiss Jonathan, because it would confirm that I was totally gay. As if rolling around with a naked man wasn't proof enough. I continued to grind against his body as if I were twelve again and had just discovered masturbation. Then, I hit the jackpot. Immediately uncomfortable, I rolled over to face the wall and stared up at a movie poster of Matt Damon a la *Good Will Hunting*. I kept hearing Robin Williams' voice in my head, "It's not all your fault. It's not all your fault."

The room was silent for a moment and finally he asked me if I was okay. My mouth remained shut, but my mind challenged, "Define okay." I had experienced my first orgasm with another person—and it was a guy. My body felt euphoric, my heart felt accepted, my brain felt ashamed, and my pride abashed; I was completely embarrassed that I came within twenty minutes of dry-humping a naked man. More humiliating still, he didn't even realize that I had climaxed until after he asked me three times if I was okay; finally reaching across the bed to feel my cargo pants covered in shame. "How do you like dem apples?"

Despite my middle school head games, my unwillingness to get naked with him, my eager ejaculation, my inexperience with sex of any kind (especially man-on-man), and my silent treatment, Jonathan rubbed my back and assured me that I had done nothing to be ashamed of.

We explored each other a few more times over the next month, me always with my pants on and Jonathan always gorgeously naked, until I went on a four month tour of Europe.

*   *   *

By the time we landed in Germany I was three sheets to the wind, only nineteen years old, my knowledge of alcohol was even less diverse than my sexual exploration. I exploited the international flight by consuming as much wine as the flight attendants could pour. It is not an exaggeration to say that I guzzled down enough wine to bankrupt a small Napa Valley start up winery.

I stood from my seat and in domino-like fashion I fell back, knocking out the two elderly Jewish men who in turn took down the line of people behind them; clearly I was in no condition to deplane, let alone find my way through an international airport and onto our tour bus without the assistance of an adult. Unwillingly one of my fellow company members stepped up to be my chaperon.

James, although only twenty-eight, had the most seniority with the company. I wouldn't describe him as traditionally handsome but he had a strong presence. He stood unusually tall for a jazz dancer. Six feet and average build with lanky arms and legs, brown hair, brown eyes, and yellow smoker's teeth. His strengths were noticeable in his ability to connect with almost everyone he met through his charming and snarky personality. He wasn't the most phenomenal dancer, but what he lacked in sparkle, he made up for in clean lines, flexibility, and effortless transitions. James was also exceptional at learning choreography quickly and retaining every step, count, and nuance. Unmistakably, he was also our company rehearsal director—a fabulous friend to have as a young apprentice with ambition.

From my very first scholarship class with the famous company, James was in my corner. Where others saw a young, green dancer with a lack of technical ability, James picked up on my drive, passion, style—and face. During my first two months at the studio he went out of his way to help me expand my technical vocabulary. It was natural that once I was promoted to a performing apprentice, he took me under his wing and continued to harness my potential.

One of the principal male dancers abruptly left the company and I jumped at the opportunity to join the ensemble on a four-month tour of Europe. Oblivious of how underprepared and inexperienced I was at the time, I led with my fearless confidence and convinced James to spend time during our rehearsal breaks to review the company repertory that I would need to know for the replacement audition. When the time came, I stood out from the rest of my peers as someone who was well versed in the pieces that we would be performing on tour. Also, I had a passport.

Now, the look of concern on James' face as he lifted me up from the aisle of the airplane made me afraid that I was in over my head. Day one into my first European tour and I was already disappointing our rehearsal director. My anxiety about traveling abroad without my family, coupled with my desire to fit in with my unreceptive cohorts, coaxed me into drowning my feelings—not a good look for a novice drinker.

We gathered our luggage, met up with our tour manager, and settled onto the bus, which would be our primary residence for the next sixteen weeks. James pulled me aside to impart some advice.

"You're not a full company member yet and you have a long road ahead of you. If you want to stay in this company, you have to take this seriously. Stay on top of your game or you won't just be hurting yourself, you'll be letting me down, too."

Point taken. Feeling the gravity of the situation I went to the back of the bus and cried. I was an amateur in Europe with performers who were older and more experienced than I. Six thousand miles away from my family—before smart phones, social media or email was easily accessible—I realized that I had to rely on the advice of James as my director and friend.

Our first performance was only three days after we arrived in Germany and I was terrified. The company arrived at the theater four hours before our call time, which gave us plenty of time to run a technical rehearsal and take a company warm-up. Moments before the curtain went up the butterflies in my stomach decided to come up and all over the bathroom floor. I sustained the first piece in our program and my nerves settled enough for me to enjoy the moment. Afterwards, I took inventory of my ability and decided that I was capable and deserving of the opportunity—otherwise I wouldn't have been hired—but I also concluded that I had tremendous work to do if I wanted to stay in the company.

On the way to our first opening night gala dinner, once again, I pulled James aside and begged him to sacrifice his spare time working with me a few evenings a week while we were on tour so that I could feel more comfortable on stage.

Whether out of concern for the company or because he just liked me, it didn't take much convincing for James to agree. We began our first rendezvous in the hallway of a German hotel that evening. Just like in the studio back in Chicago, James assumed his position as rehearsal director and began reviewing the counts of choreography, stopping occasionally to adjust my arms or give me a correction on style. Unlike in the studio, he was more playful and flirtatious.

I brushed off his innuendo as "locker room shenanigans" in order to pass the time while working on tedious material. He knew that I was straight (or more factually, he knew that I was deep in the closet, but maintained that I was straight), so I didn't worry about his harmless humor. He was sacrificing his time off in Europe to help me; the least I could do was throw him a bone. If only it had occurred to me then, that when you give a gay a bone, they get a boner.

The late night sessions in the hallways of random hotels across Europe continued and our level of intimacy increased as well. James was generous with his time, and even in my naïve state, it was clear that his feelings for me were shifting from mentor to a man who might want more. I began confiding in him things that I hadn't talked about with anyone else and I felt safe that he wouldn't betray my trust.

By our second week in Germany I was starting to feel comfortable, both on stage and off, with the rest of my peers. I had discovered a new depth to my confidence as a person and dancer in large part thanks to the coaching and counseling that James had provided. Not all of the company members were convinced that I was a suitable replacement, only now it didn't matter. James was in my camp and our evening escapades evolved from casual choreography coaching in the hallways of hotels into a nightly slumber party in his room.

It wasn't like *that,* at first. There was no touching involved, primarily because each of us had a female roommate on the road.*

James, Sandra (his roommate), and I would sit up until three in the morning sharing our dreams, bitching about the other company members, and binge eating Ritter Sport chocolate bars. Eventually, Sandra would pretend to doze off, and James and I would continue our revealing conversation. Most of the things he would divulge were about his childhood and being gay. I wasn't an idiot, I realized that he was trying to entice me to come out, but I was not ready to take the bait. I was ready to masturbate though—and so the touching began.

I was starting to find my groove with the company and my work on stage was beginning to blossom. One evening, after my best performance to date, I expressed my gratitude to James. We were lying on his bed (above the covers) and I was still pumped full of adrenaline. Sandra was fast asleep when James reached over and

---

* Our artistic director was a firm believer that we should share a hotel room with the opposite sex to reduce the drama. Ironically, we were paired with our primary dance partner so that whatever fight or calamity we encountered on stage could continue in the hotel room after the show.

started massaging my back. I was nervous at first; unlike with Mark and Jonathan, I was not physically attracted to James. I caved to his gentle, supportive touch, and granted access toward my inner thigh. Soon, I was under the covers and rolling around with James. Again, I found a way to control my situation; no kissing and my underwear remained on, which proved a challenge for his hands.

We made our way across Europe dancing on stage by day and in the sheets at night. We never spoke about what was happening and we tried to hide it from the other company members, but the subtle glances and off-the-cuff comments that James would make on our tour bus encouraged inquisitions.

The fact that my roommate had a hotel room to herself should have been the first clue; thankfully she was busy having an affair of her own with our pot-smoking tour manager Klaus.

I did my best to shield against the rumors and accusations, until one night—halfway through our European tour—the company decided to investigate the nightlife in Berlin. Klaus suggested a popular discothèque in the heart of the city.

Nineteen years old and in a foreign country without my mom or dad, surrounded by hot, sweaty European men and women dancing to Cher. "Do you believe in life after love?" Yes, Cher, as a matter of fact, I do. And to prove it, I managed to get lost in a corner of the pulsing nightclub, pinned against a wall by yet another company member whom I was on tour with, Billy. Billy looked like a young George Michael. His body came close to me in slow motion, his lips were on mine and his tongue had twisted itself around mine. My heart pounded a harmonious percussion as my body experienced a rush of heat and tingling that I imagine felt like the perfect dose of heroine. I was in lust and because I was in Berlin (and incredibly drunk) I didn't care about the rules I had spent my entire life obeying.

Just as fast as I had allowed the embrace to happen, I decidedly forced the Mardi-Gras-make-out session to an end.

Courtney Love-drunk, we stumbled our way through the streets of Berlin, onto a train and back to the hotel, not before (in true American arrogance) getting kicked off of a statue erected near a portion of the former Berlin Wall that we'd climbed for a photo-op.

Once we arrived at the hotel it was decided that the party should continue in one of our hotel rooms, and because I was the youngest—

and paired with a female roommate who was always ready for booze, boys, and all things bad—the night raged on.

Like a Hollywood sex-scandal leaked by TMZ, Billy exposed our headline news. James was visibly shaken, but thankfully he did not confront me in the moment. Before I knew it, we were playing Truth or Dare and I was entirely sure whom everyone was coming for.

Around the same time Klaus decided to break out the bud. Apparently this would be a night of firsts for me! The geographical and sociological distance between Europe and the United States, teamed with the European nonchalance toward taboo subjects, and my yearning to be less calculated and more carefree, gave me permission to intrude on my boundaries and abandon my issues with trust.

Klaus loaded up the bong and started passing it around the room as I began to challenge two things: Should I smoke pot? And should I tell everyone that I thought I was gay? Both, burdensome questions to be asking myself in the current state of mind, no matter how I answered they would impact the rest of my life. I suddenly felt like a child.

Mirroring events that transpired earlier in the evening, the bong was passed to me and my lips were introduced to a new object. I was inhaling "the best bud you'll ever have" according to Klaus. (Which was and remains to be true at the time of publishing this book.) I sat back and felt a calm overcome me. Never in my life had I found such a peace of mind. Without the inner monologue that normally ruled my thoughts, I was able to not-give-a-shit. In under five minutes I was up and entertaining the entire room.

I have always been someone who was eager to get a laugh, primarily to distract from facing reality—like a magician, I was ready to smash my inner dove for the sake of applause. High and carefree I was acting out sketches I'd seen on Saturday Night Live in order to refocus my colleagues' attention from my gay tendencies. And it worked.

Later, during our tour, another openly gay performer in our group cornered me and decided to give me a palm reading. He was a dancer who freelanced as a fortune teller. He explained that he only had the ability when "called to bring clarity to someone in need". This time, rather than a seductive kiss, I was getting an earful of things I already knew with a dash of the obvious.

All gay men will attest: we can spot a closet case from the opposite side of the Universe. And no, we don't think every hot male celebrity is undoubtedly gay—only the ones who sleep with men.

What my psychic experience did reveal is that: A.) I was NOT ready to deal with coming out, and B.) I WILL be successful in the entertainment industry, but fortune and fame wouldn't come until I was in my forties.*

Four months, five countries, twenty cities, thirty performances, and plenty of "life experience" later, our European tour was coming to an end.

James waited for the perfect opportunity to corner me on the back of the tour bus in order to "clarify" our relationship. I knew that I would eventually have to deal with the consequences of hooking up with my rehearsal director on tour; I had hoped that moment would come privately. Not speeding down the autobahn with a bus full of my peers.

The initial confrontation was tough. It was indisputable that James was more invested (in love) with me than I was with him. I remained totally transparent during the course of our entire SEXperiment; the proverb, "actions speak louder than words" suddenly made sense.

I had been honest, albeit very selfish. Emotionally, we mutually confided about our past, our fears, our dreams, and coming to terms with our sexuality. Physically, I never reciprocated; James did all of the touching and I did all of the feeling.

Our conversation went back and forth until I declared that I was in no way ready to "come out". Like our time on tour, I professed that our inappropriate touching would be ending. He accused me of using him and I retaliated by claiming that he abused my trust.

The ten-hour airplane ride back to Chicago was somber. The exhilaration of performing with a world-renowned dance company across Europe was overshadowed by a sex-scandal. I could officially relate to a Bill Clinton.

Fact: The Gay Mafia does exist. Within thirty minutes of my arrival at O'Hare airport, most of the Chicagoland area knew that my manhood was up for grabs.

I could not yet face the thought of my friends (or GOD FORBID) my family finding out. Worse yet was facing my best friend, Kristen.

---

* I am a happily married gay man, and I just turned forty—so I'm really hoping that the second half of my reading comes true!

Prior to leaving town she had expressed strong feelings for me. We had shared a few tender nights cuddling, but I knew there was an expectation of heavy petting upon my return.

Similar to what you'd expect in an early 1990's independent film now airing on the Sundance Channel, the minute I returned stateside I created an alter ego in order to cope with the fallout of my overseas transgressions. In a desperate attempt to fast track my sexual orientation status and appease my eager roommate (Oh, did I mention that Kristen was also my roommate?), I complicated matters by having sex with her two days after returning to Chicago.

I masturbated a lot, but sex was never something I would let myself think about growing up. At the time, I told myself that I needed to pour all of my energy into following my dreams. In my head, it made sense that losing my virginity should happen with someone I loved—if not physically then emotionally. In actuality, I was fighting the inevitable.

There were a handful of people who knew the truth about what happened on tour and then there was everyone who had heard a version of the truth.

James was obviously distraught and spent the first two weeks vacillating between anger and hate, and then compassion and pity. He was still my rehearsal director, thus he held a power over me, which he used in rehearsals. We had spent nearly four months together sharing vulnerabilities, now he was exposing my flaws—publically.

Kristen heard the rumors from many of the company members who befriended her only after the news of our romance began. Had Facebook existed at the time, my status would have shifted from "single" to "it's complicated", but the social media machine was ten years too late; so Kristen relied on her intuition. She never asked me if the rumors were true and I never spoke about my time on the road. She was one of the first people I met when I moved to Chicago and had been my closest companion. She was also privy to my earlier indiscretions with Mark and Jonathan. Neither of which seemed to concern her at the time. I believe Kristen saw the potential for a promising future with me. She witnessed my drive, trusted in my passion, and affixed herself to my ambition; in doing so, she overlooked the fundamental flaw in our perfect love story.

After three years in Chicago, I decided that it was time to escape my past and expand my career in New York City. Kristen's bags were packed before I asked her if she was coming.

Denial is an interesting defense mechanism. If you embody your lie deeply enough to live in it fully, it becomes the truth that others are forced to accept. I was so desperate to be the cool, confident, handsome, straight man with a movie star career, a wife, two children, a dog, and a home in the Hollywood Hills. Kristen wanted that dream for me—for us—and became my willing accomplice.

Jingle Bell Cock

Part I: Unraveling

Everyone in the cast knew our dirty little secret, even before we did. The beginning of an innocent friendship that would ultimately lead to the permanent unraveling of the shameful lie I spent my entire life living. Deceiving family, friends, and worst of all—myself, into a twenty-two year game of charades, I was finally ready to come out of the closet; and on what better occasion than while dancing in the ensemble of the largest (and quite possibly gayest) Christmas Spectacular on the planet.

On our first day of rehearsal, all of the newly-hired cast members were greeted with a wretched amount of information. We were thrown into a twelve-hour, military-style boot camp of learning choreography, music, and stage directions that would have made Ebenezer Scrooge drop a load of coal in his long underwear. By lunch I was in desperate search of a safe place to cry, like a child who's just seen the Grinch.

As I was making my way down the long hallway from the rehearsal studio into our lounge, I hallucinated a small herd of reindeer, which turned out to be new chorus members who were just as dazed and confused as I was. Ready to abandon the building as soon as possible, I suggested that we all go grab lunch at Rockefeller Center—the fresh air would do us all good; even in a state of panic and despair I was always ready to meet new people (and eat).

We sat and watched the ice skaters blissfully twirl around the rink pretending to be Tara Lipinski, as we somberly ate our food, until finally I decided that someone had to break the ice and it might as well be me. Rather than revealing my true panic, I decided to casually joke about how intense the rehearsal process was. "Well, it was nice to get to know all of you, even for one day. They told me there was no need to return after lunch, apparently Santa thinks I'm doing a bad job."

As soon as the words left my lips, the intensity at the table went from mild terror to Stresscon-10.

"Wait, they're firing you on our first day?" Someone in my new Christmas clique asked.

"No, but it sure feels like we're all under an extreme microscope doesn't it?"

With that, a breath of holiday air warmed the atmosphere and we began to really talk shop. One after another, people began to expose their fears, allowing us to form a bond that would help us maneuver through the (literal) camel shit that was still in store for us during our run.

Shortly following that lunch, I became close with one of the other newbies in the male ensemble. Daniel was the textbook definition of a male dancer: he stood six feet tall, his narrow waist led a perfect trail upward to his sleek yet muscular torso, his Euro-handsome face and lustrous jet-black hair sat strong on his V-lined shoulders and arms that simultaneously proclaimed strength and comfort. His well-defined legs were shadowed with the perfect amount of hair, and his feet had an arch that would make a banana jealous. His technique and ability as a dancer and performer matched perfectly with his ridiculous physique. If it were possible, you would believe he was the love child of Keanu Reeves (the early years) and Baryshnikov—everyone wanted to *know* Daniel.

As I stood in line waiting for my turn to rehydrate at the water cooler, Daniel approached me and offered Altoids—never one to shy away from fresh breath, I gladly accepted. As I reached for the fresh-mouth-maker, I was so nervous that I knocked the entire tin of mints onto the floor. He looked down and with a goofy face he looked up and said, "If that's the way you feel about fresh breath, I'm concerned."

I was hooked on Daniel like a stay-at-home-parent is to prescription pills. From that point on we became inseparable, which was very easy during our grueling rehearsal schedule. We spent twelve-hour days learning combinations, running sections of the show, and continually proving our worthiness as performers. Between breaks and after rehearsals, Daniel and I would check in with one another, and occasionally we would go out for drinks to blow off steam. After nearly two weeks of random conversations about nothing and small talk, we elevated our level of friendship by opening up about our personal life.

I finally revealed that I was in a serious relationship with a girl who I had moved to New York with and that we were planning on getting married. Why it had taken me so long to share this information was beyond my grasp. Even more explosive was the discovery that Daniel was also in a long-term relationship with a woman, which he saved until this moment to divulge.

Instead of calling it a night and returning home to our insignificant others, we ordered up another round of dirty Martinis from the attractive bartender who had been keeping a close account of our nightly conversations. Without actually admitting anything (yet), Daniel and I had broken through a barrier that we'd both lived behind for so long. We identified with each other and it was now safe to speak freely to one-another without fear of being caught or judged. He became the only person I could trust completely, which was gratifying and guilt-inducing all at the same time. As the rehearsal process continued, I would eagerly await our post-work day cocktails; during which we shared our darkest fears, most ambitious goals, and deepest desires.

We would talk until our bartender, James (with whom we were now on a first name basis and who was openly flirting with both of us) would make last call, at which point we had no choice but to return home to our manufactured lives with girlfriends included. Eventually my girlfriend demanded to know why I never invited her out to meet my cast, and I explained that until this moment everyone had been too overwhelmed to meet new people.

The next morning on my walk to the theater, I decided to plan a group outing with my Christmas crew in order to introduce them to the much-hyped-but-still-elusive girlfriend. Once I'd come clean to Daniel, I spent most of my days at rehearsal talking about her out of a lifelong habit to be perceived as a hetero-performer.

The introductions went as expected—my girlfriend, Kristen, was beautiful and unafraid to be herself. My castmates connected their own dots and we ordered margaritas. I strategically chose Arriba Arriba (a popular Mexican restaurant among the theater crowd) for their delicious drinks and the loud atmosphere; lively conversation and schoolgirl gossip ensued. Toward the end of the evening, Kristen decided that she should interrogate Daniel—thankfully the rest of our cast had stumbled home to prepare for our dress rehearsal the next day (also a calculated move on my part).

After a rapid-fire line of invasive questions and mild attacks on Daniel's character, Kristen was convinced that we were nothing more than close friends who enjoyed venting with a few drinks after slaving in Santa's workshop all day.

I woke up the next morning ready to face the most exciting day of my New York experience as a performer. After weeks of rehearsals, costume fittings, and animal training (where we learned how to tame our sheep and walk around camel dung) our final dress rehearsal with a full audience was upon us. Performing on the stage at Radio City Music Hall is unlike anything I've ever experienced before or after. There are over sixty members of the cast, twenty dressers (who manage to quick change the entire cast in under thirty seconds), a full orchestra, a Living Nativity, six animal handlers (who live in the basement), and no spectacular would be complete without six little people dressed as elves. All things considered, I thought our first full run of the show went exceedingly well. Unfortunately, our director and the trusty team of producers felt otherwise, and the two-hour note session began.

With less than an ounce of dignity remaining, our cast quickly made their way to the unofficial cast party (the official cast party wasn't scheduled until opening night) but you can always count on "show people" to plan events around alcohol—especially after the lackluster review we just received from the ~~Dictator~~, director.

Sitting at the bar alongside Daniel was Val, another close friend I made during the rehearsal process. Val was a vibrant, fun-loving woman who actually enjoyed my exuberant personality and sassy stage presence. She lovingly gave me the nickname "LA", referring to my colorful energy and boyish good looks.

I gently forced myself between Val and Daniel and interjected my unsolicited thoughts about our run through. Daniel excused himself to the restroom, and Val took this opportunity to begin a conversation that felt like something you might hear from Roma Downey in a Hallmark special.

"I want you to know that I am here for you, and love you unconditionally. I think you are a bright star, and I know that you will go so far in life. And if you ever need to talk [long uncomfortable pause] about anything at all [another gratuitous pause] I. Am. Here. For. You."

"Thanks Val, that means a lot to me."

"I'm serious. I don't know where your girlfriend is, but I imagine you didn't invite her for a reason, and no one is judging you for that."

"Should they be?" I began to sweat.

"Well, look around. It's an important night, and everyone else is standing with his or her loved one. It seems Kristen doesn't really support you."

"Oh, it's not that at all... She had to work, and I didn't really think this was such a big deal," I lied.

"Well, regardless, if you need to talk, I'm here for you. I can keep a secret. Oh, and if you should find yourself in need of a place to stay, a very close friend of mine is looking for a roommate, and you two would hit it off perfectly!"

With that, Val gave me a kiss on the cheek and headed off to mingle with the cast.

When I got back to my apartment that evening, I felt ashamed that I had not asked Kristen to join me in celebrating with my cast. I climbed into bed and stared off into the darkness, contemplating how on Earth I was going to deal with all of *this*. Sure, there had been many sleepless nights toiling over how, or if, I was ever going to allow myself to act on these feelings that (if I'm being honest) I had felt since I was in third grade—but for some reason that night I realized I was finally ready to come clean with my LIFE.

If Facebook had existed back then coming out might have been completely different, but without it, how do you confront almost everyone you've come in contact with to tell them, "Okay, you were right—I am gay and I just couldn't deal with it until now." Unsure of how to proceed, I concentrated all of my energy on the show and rationalized that everything would work out eventually.

Part II: The Reveal

Firmly in the middle of our run, Daniel and I were closer than ever. While the rest of the male ensemble would carry on in the dressing room between shows, we would sneak off into a stairwell between the third and fourth floors of Radio City Music Hall to bond. Our non-sexual encounters were filled with philosophical conversations, writing in our journals, and me gazing into Daniel's eyes, while he practiced playing his guitar and serenading me with *Mr. Jones* by the Counting Crows. It couldn't get any gayer than that—even if we *were* having sex.

As Christmas approached I was spending very little time at home and entirely too much time with Daniel. One evening after a long show day, Daniel and I decided to grab some food before calling it a night. At first glance, our dinner was nothing out of the ordinary. The conversation was stimulating and intoxicating—that was the magical aspect of Daniel, he made everyone feel special when he talked. Upon closer examination it was obvious that between every playful innuendo the sexual tension was building in correlation to the number of drinks we consumed that night. When spirits rise, so do other things. Eager to get outside and extinguish the fire burning in my crotch, I reached for the check before we could even discuss *dessert*.

We exited the restaurant on 5th Avenue and 51st Street, which is always romantic during the holidays, and decided that it was the perfect night to walk the twenty-plus blocks and through Central Park to get home. Neither of us was in a hurry to abandon the company of the other, and we'd each consumed three fishbowls full of a bright neon alcohol that was sure to keep our bones warm.

Just as we crossed the South East entrance to Central Park it began to snow. We followed the winding path past The Pond, around Wollman Rink and over to the Sheep's Meadow. The night was so quiet we could hear the snowflakes land on our eyelashes. We glanced back to savor the skyline of Manhattan glistening through the falling powder—it was a living Currier and Ives winter wonderland.

Daniel turned to me, "Mattie, can I tell you something."

My heart was beating nervously as I stammered, "Of course."

"I think I like you."

Now, despite the frost in the air, my heart was melting, "I like you, too."

"No, I mean, I like you in a way that I'm not supposed to."

"Yes, Daniel, I understood that—I have the same feeling inside. I've been trying to figure out how to tell you for a while."

He smiled, playfully rubbed the back of my head, and asked if we could hold hands; without waiting for an answer he reached down and took my hand into his and we continued to walk in silence toward Central Park West.

Even through our gloves the electricity was flowing. A trillion thoughts, fears, and emotions raced through my head simultaneously as my *other* head was filling with blood.

We approached the exit and I knew our moment was going to come to an end. I was trying to convince myself to do the right thing—continue walking three blocks back to my apartment and face my girlfriend—instead, Daniel hailed a cab and we climbed in.

As the cab drove up Central Park West our handholding transitioned into a softcore Taxi Cab confession make-out session. At last, Daniel's tongue was one with mine. His strong hands applied pressure on the back of my head pulling me into him. The stubble of his beard and the woodsy scent of his Canadian manhood aroused my body in a way that I had never encountered. We came up for air just in time to see our not so subtly off-put taxi cab driver pull up to Daniel's apartment.

Safely upstairs and in the warmth of Daniel's candlelit room, he turned on Sade—for someone who'd never hooked up with a guy before he sure knew what he was doing.

We sat at the edge of his futon mattress and stared at each other, both unsure of what would come next. Our naked feet initiated the next phase of sexual exploration as Sade whispered sensual encouragement.

After forty minutes of teenage-like dry humping, my heart was conflicted and my penis was raw. I felt terrible that I didn't feel guilty about what was happening; while Kristen was at home waiting for me, I was falling in love for the first time. I pushed Daniel off me, explaining that I had to resolve my conflict with Kristen. At once I had the confidence to say out loud that I was gay, and I had to do so before my conviction disappeared. I grabbed my things and headed toward Columbus Avenue. I spent the entire fifteen-minute walk replaying the last three hours. I had no idea what I was going to say to Kristen, but I knew that there was no turning back—I tasted the fruit, literally, and I was hooked.

I arrived at our apartment just after three o'clock in the morning, took a deep breath and opened the door. There was no hiding from the truth as I stepped into the 200 square foot room we called our home—the lights were blazing and Kristen sat in the middle of our bed, wide-awake and ready to attack. I felt like a politician involved in a sex-scandal going to face the media for the first time, only I knew a camera lens would have been much less invasive then the interrogation that was about to proceed.

I could feel the chill of Kristen's bitterness the moment I dropped my backpack by the door, took off my winter layers and sat at the edge of the bed.

Then it began. "Where have you been? I've been up all night waiting for you. You were out with *him*, weren't you?"

"I don't even know where to start."

"Just tell me what's going on."

"Well, you know I love you—I really do. You've been my best friend, you support my decisions and you can make me laugh harder than anyone I know..."

"You don't love me anymore?"

"Kristen, I'm gay. I think we've both always known this—and I really wanted to marry you, and have a family and be rich and famous. I just, I don't know how to keep doing this. I can't keep living a lie."

My ears went numb and started ringing—then a complete silence filled the room. Kristen's face was fire engine red as she broke the silence, screaming at the top of her lungs, "Your family is going to HATE you. You aren't going to have any friends. You will never make it as an actor and I will never speak to you again. I can't believe you lied to me."

"I know you're angry and you don't understand. Believe me, I can't really process this either. I've just reached a point where all of those things that you said might be true and I don't care—I *can't* care— anymore. I've spent too much time worrying about hiding this feeling. Agonizing whether my dreams will crumble if I'm honest with who I am and what I feel inside; and I guess I've just reached a point where my *life* means more to me. I hope you can understand this."

Kristen was calculated. "I cheated on you twice and I never felt bad about it because I knew deep down you would do this to me one day."

Kristen's confession came as no surprise to me. I'd discovered her first infidelity accidentally through a friend. After a night of drinking and dancing, a mutual friend encouraged me to flirt with a guy at an after-hours party. When I reminded my friend that I was *straight* and in a relationship with his close friend, he laughed and told me that she had cheated on me with a Northwestern University football star.

Finding out about the second affair was stinging—but I was not in a place to dredge up the past. I was finally able to unmask my inner self, my true identity, and I didn't care about anything other than peacefully moving forward. I looked at Kristen and apologized for hurting her.

Suddenly a calm energy engulfed the room. Kristen was quiet—we stared each other in the eyes and began to cry. I had destroyed her illusion of me, and the life that we worked so hard to achieve together.

I did my best to explain that my love was never a lie. I sincerely loved Kristen and I wanted to be the man that she expected, needed, believed I was—but I knew that my feelings for her were different than her love for me.

I reached out and gave her a hug. We held on to one another for a long embrace, and then I pulled away. I had to let go or there was no hope of convincing her that this was real. Kristen had a way of manipulating me into doing things I knew I shouldn't. If I stayed a minute longer I would have given in to her appeal.

I can assure you that there is no "right time" to come out, but I can fully admit that two weeks before Christmas is less than ideal. I promised Kristen that I would pay the rent for the following three months, giving her plenty of time to find a new place or roommate. We didn't own much in our pint-sized apartment, but I assured her that she could keep anything that she wanted. I packed a bag of clothing and threw in a few of my personal effects, journals, and sentimental objects and told her I'd come back to collect the rest of my things when she was at work.

I took another long deep breath. "You have been my best friend and I'm so sorry that our story is ending like this. Thank you for the love, laughter, and support that you have shared with me. I hope that one day you will forgive me. Whether that day comes or not, I wish nothing but the best for you." As I closed the door and walked down the hallway I felt a sense of relief. It took every bit of strength to turn my back on the world that I had created, but that fabrication was now in my past. Without pause, I jumped in a cab and headed back to Daniel's apartment. He was waiting with more sensual soft rock and open arms. I was reborn and I wasn't going to look back.

Part III: Born Again

The show on the Great Stage the following day was less of a Spectacular and more like a spectacle; rumor of my "Gigantic Fat Gay Break-Up" spread like an STD in a bathhouse. Suddenly everyone in the cast thought it was okay to laugh about how obvious it was that I was GAY.

I effervescently made my way down 6th Avenue toward the 51st Stage Door entrance ready to start my new life. Immediately inside the male ensemble dressing room I was engulfed by flames from shady, jaded, chorus-boys who sat in silence as their eyes stared me up and down with "I always knew it" judgment. I thought gay men were overjoyed when exuberant, youthful, physically fit closet-casers came out? (Now, many years later, I've realized that just like witches in OZ there are good gays and bad.)

Somehow the entire men's dressing room had figured out that I had broke up with my girlfriend. I had no idea who clued them in, and I didn't care to find out. I rushed into my first costume and headed down to the stage earlier than normal to avoid any unpleasant confrontations.

Once down on the stage I was met with a similar air of awkwardness from the stagehands and crew, until one of my straight buddies in the crew came over and shook my hand and offered me an honest congratulations. Following that much needed *hand job*, the crew smiled and they continued setting the stage as normal. I stood panicked in a wing stage left and watched as ensemble members and Rockettes made their way onto the stage. When the lights went dim and the orchestra began playing the overture, I made my way to my mark.

I never visualized what it would look like if I grew the balls to finally come out; now I'm balling my eyes out in a giant panda bear costume during the Nutcracker scene, because someone outed me on my special day. With a heavy heart, I accepted that I was robbed of my coming out moment—worse yet, the men in the ensemble didn't even give me my gay card.

By the last scene in act one, I was on the verge of a meltdown. The Rockettes were grouped like models in a storefront window display. I was hand in hand with my dance partner Akemi, a beautiful Japanese dancer who spoke no English, pretending to window shop. I was reluctant to continue with our choreography because one of the Rockettes in the next faux window display was a dear friend of mine who also happened to be my ex-girlfriend's best friend. I hadn't talked to her since our break-up and I had no idea if I was losing her in the separation. Akemi could feel my hesitance and nudged me to begin the traffic pattern that we were now two counts late starting. We approached the window and I saw Amber posed with the same gorgeous smile as always. Ordinarily this was an instance in the show where I would break character (facing upstage of course) and pull faces in order to get the Rockettes to break their perfect mannequin character.

Instead, Amber locked eyes with me, smiled bigger and gave me a wink. My eyes welled up and then the years of bottled up emotions and present joy spilled all over the stage. Akemi broke character for the first time on stage asking, "Are you okay?" I couldn't respond, I just continued crying—White Christmas in New York came to life in a way that I had never experienced before. I was awake.

In the middle of Santa's workshop, one of the gay little people (dressed as an elf) walked up to me and said, "Congratulations! Welcome to the rest of your life, it's like Christmas every day!"

I took inventory of the massive stage, where I was surrounded by a cast of crazy people who play dress-up and pretend for a living. It occurred to me that they weren't judging me, they were applauding me for coming clean.

As for the dressing room afterwards, most of the male ensemble approached me and shared their coming out story. It was reassuring to hear how others had lived through similar situations. They offered advice, support and (some) their phone numbers. Suddenly it dawned on me why they were so quiet before the show. My newfound homosexuality reminded them of their own struggles coming to terms with the lies they endured before coming out. No matter how unique our version is—it's a bond we all share.

Part IV: Rebuilding

I was liberated and fearless—like I could conquer the world, which I soon discovered I might actually have to do. Logistically speaking I had so much to figure out. Where would I live? How will I tell my family? WHAT am I going to do about my tragically unfashionable clothing? I was always very well styled for a straight guy, but no respectable gay New Yorker would be caught dead in fleece.

The housing situation was under control thanks to my fortune telling friend Val. She approached me the day after my sexuality exploded on the world's largest stage: "Hey LA, I wanted to let you know that my friend Cathy still has that room available. I called her this morning and she's expecting a call from you."

I called Cathy and scheduled to meet her for coffee at the apartment after our matinee. As I walked across town toward Hell's Kitchen, I decided to stop at an ATM and withdraw $500.00. I hadn't even seen the apartment, but I trusted Val and her taste in friends, I loved the desirable midtown location, and I knew that I couldn't go through the drama of searching for an apartment. I was taking this place regardless of its condition, and nothing sets a "good roommate tone" better than showing up with cash.

Sure enough, Cathy and I hit it off from her perfectly timed gay joke and opening hug. She was ten years my senior, which was ideal, and she had a similar family background—we shared a common Catholic guilt.

After swapping our life stories, Cathy gave me a tour of the apartment, which didn't take long. It was what New Yorkers affectionately referred to as a shotgun apartment, because with one shot you could hit someone in every room of the house, and all this goodness could be mine for just five-hundred and fifty dollars a month. Cathy had only two rules: no smoking and no overnight guests. I was sold. I dropped the cash onto the kitchen table and told her I'd bring the $50.00 balance tomorrow when I moved in!

I had the quintessential coming-out-of-the-closet sized roof over my head. Now, how to deal with my family? I thought about sending personalized notes with glitter enclosed, but that felt too flamboyant and coming out over the phone felt too impersonal. Because this was my first big show in New York City, my mom and her husband, Steve, had planned to visit over Christmas, which was only a week away. I decided I would come out to them first, because they had always been the most open and I would determine a plan of attack based on their reaction.

I greeted my family a week later. I wasted no time explaining to them that Kristin and I had broken up, but left the details very vague.

That night after my show I asked my parents if I could invite a friend out to dinner with us. Daniel and I headed up Central Park West toward the Empire Hotel and met my family for dinner at Pomodoro's Italian restaurant on the Upper West Side.

After brief introductions we jumped right into a thoughtful conversation about family and friends where Daniel effortlessly charmed my mom and bonded with Steve. After our second glass of wine I started reenacting ridiculous sketches that I was working on in my acting class, which prompted laughter from all, and an unconscious vote of support from Daniel. The pat of praise on my left thigh happened quickly under the table and under the radar, so I thought.

After dinner Steve suggested that we get back to the hotel to get some sleep in preparation for a full day of Christmas mayhem. We said our goodbyes to Daniel and walked back to the hotel. As we passed through the lobby my mom and Steve paused, exchanged glances and then asked me to join them for a drink in the hotel bar. I was already tipsy, wide-awake and drunk on love—naturally I obliged.

Steve ordered dirty Martinis all around. Upgrading to the clear booze, I was not sure where this impromptu Christmas Eve was headed.

We clinked drinks and invited the live jazzy holiday music to ease us into Christmas. After a strange pause, my mom turned to me and said, "Matthew, I'm so proud of you son. You're following your dreams. You know I will always love you, and you can tell me anything right?"

"Thanks, mom. I love you, too. I'm so grateful for your support."

Steve chimed in, "We just love you so much and we want you to be happy no matter what path you take in life."

Suddenly I felt a panic in my bowels—you know, the feeling you get in high school when you have to change in the locker room next to the captain of the football team, who also happens to be the only guy in tenth grade buying (and using) Magnum condoms.

"Thanks guys. You've been so supportive of my dreams." (I started to cry.) *This is my moment—what am I afraid of? They just told me they'd love me no matter what.*

"Matt, are you gay?" Steve asked without warning in a compassionate tone.

"Yes." I erupted into a full-blown Pageant Queen victory sob. It felt so satisfying to be free of that guilt, shame, and embarrassment. The unconditional love I experienced was priceless.

My mom proclaimed her gaydar: "I knew the moment Daniel grabbed your leg at dinner that you two were a *thing*. I've always known really—you've always cared so much about fashion, style, and cologne."

"A *thing?*" I laughed. "If you always knew, why didn't you ask me?"

"I don't know. Your dad and I talked about it a few times while you were growing up. I guess we just assumed you would tell us eventually. Then once you started dating girls we just thought you'd figured it out."

"Dad knows?"

"Well, not officially. Unless you told your sister and she told him."

"No, you and Steve are the only people in our family who know. I want to tell everyone in person."

"Well, I wouldn't keep it from your dad or sister too long, you know how fast these things spread. Make sure they hear it from you before they're caught off guard by someone else."

We finished our second Martini and headed up to the hotel room. I slept better that night than I had since I was a child. It was a Christmas miracle.

I had two shows on Christmas Day, so we woke up early and headed out for a day of shopping on 5th Avenue. My mom suggested that I update my wardrobe to better complement my newfound fabulousness.

Words you never thought you'd want to hear from your mom: "Those are the perfect pants for you. They really accentuate your cute butt."

Three hours, twenty stores, two credit cards, and six bags full of designer duds that screamed controversial (before metrosexual was a word) and my costume change was complete. I was now fully prepared to rule my new gay life.

Mom and Steve's visit continued with more food, shopping, shows, cocktails—and tales of cock (my mom was not afraid to hear the *meaty* truth about my new lifestyle).

Alas, I was fresh on the scene and had very little scandal for her to sink her teeth into. I stood on the corner of Broadway and 66th and waved goodbye to the yellow cab that carried them back to Colorado. I looked down at my burgundy snakeskin Kenneth Cole loafers and matching saddlebag (which was very on point at the time) and chuckled; once I embrace something, I really go all out.

With astounding approval, my cast was fast to react to my overnight homo-makeover. Suddenly I walked and talked more confidently.

Part V: The Betrayal

By mid April, Daniel and I had spent countless hours together soul searching and planning our future. One day over coffee with a group of friends he mentioned that his parents were arriving from Canada later in the day for a visit. I was thrown by this news. I didn't understand why he waited so long to tell me, and why he chose to do so in front of some random friends.

From my perplexed reaction Daniel offered a last minute invitation to dinner at our favorite vegetarian restaurant, Zen Palate. I accepted the invitation noting that I was now that girl who gets asked to the prom only after the guy's first ten choices turn him down.

I arrived early to ensure a stellar first impression. Daniel and his mom and dad were waiting in the lounge area. In a very formal way, Daniel introduced me to his mom and dad. He omitted the words "gay", "dating", and "love". But included the words "buddy" and "good guy".

We were seated soon after and wasted no time with small talk. Daniel's father was intelligent and insightful; he conducted conversation like we were musicians in the New York Philharmonic.

After a somber discussion over the lack of career opportunities for this generation we eased into our second course of "clean eating" with soy-based meatless Chinese fare and our conversation shifted into a more personal exchange.

I opened up about my background and gained a few laughs (and the approval of Daniel's mother) with some of my outlandish teenage dramas. I started to feel safe and open—ready to share my latest discovery, I felt Daniel's foot reprimand my shin from under the table. Just like that, I was being kicked back into the closet in front of our tofu orange chicken.

Back at Daniel's apartment I sat furious and brokenhearted. I didn't understand why the evening was so inauthentic. "What happened?"

"Mattie, my parents don't know I'm gay, and I don't think I will ever be able to tell them."

I couldn't believe the words I was hearing. Is this the same guy who held my hand in Central Park under the stunning moonlight? "What do you mean? They seemed like completely reasonable and loving people—I'm sure they'll support you. I bet they already know."

"They are wonderful parents. I love them and I know they love me. But they would never accept me if I were gay. There's a side that they don't show many people. I grew up in a very Catholic home, and they expect me to lead a moral life."

Before long spring had warmed its way into New York City and the uncomfortable tension between Daniel and me had cooled. I was feeling more confident in my sexuality while simultaneously developing an unhealthy dependency on Daniel. It wasn't long before he suggested that we spend more time away from one another to establish ourselves as openly gay men. For Daniel, this meant dating other guys, although he didn't tell me that at the time.

I was heading down 9th Avenue to meet up with a friend for lunch. Two blocks away from the café I noticed a good-looking man with dark hair. At first I was proud of myself for feeling secure enough to check out a guy in public without fear of being caught, but as I got closer my body began to tremble. I could feel my heart trying to squeeze its way out of my body via my butt hole. I clinched my cheeks as tears streamed uncontrollably down my face.

Daniel was walking hand in hand with another guy. The next ten minutes felt like I was in a motion capture film—I jumped behind a box of fruit outside of a bodega. I peered my head around the bananas to get a closer look at this guy. He was tall and stocky with salt and pepper hair. I caught a glimpse of his profile as he was reacting to something Daniel was saying, and I noticed that his face looked to be mid thirties. This was no friend of Daniel's that I'd ever met. Daniel was clearly on a date. Why would he choose a spot in Hell's Kitchen only two blocks away from my apartment? Did he want me to find out?

As dignified as one can be, hiding behind a palate of fruit in Hell's Kitchen, I pulled myself together and re-routed myself to lunch. When I arrived, my friend could see that I was out of sorts and did her best to comfort me.

Daniel and I had previously made plans to meet up for coffee and a journaling session that evening, so I decided to press an emotional pause button and go into full-blown hysteria once my suspicions were confirmed.

The evening was strained to say the least. For no apparent reason (to him) I gave him the cold shoulder and used less than ten words in the first hour of our Zen time. I come from a family of hot-headed Italians who are used to shouting everything—if you want to express love, you yell it from across the room—so it took the strength of a Kardsashian's Spanx to stay calm and casually mention the encounter.

He shared his feelings, and I cried. I shared my feelings, and I cried some more. Daniel was honest and I had to accept that he was exploring his sexuality, too. If he wanted to go on a date with an older, less attractive, small business owner from Long Island—who was I to stand in his way?

That night was a turning point in our relationship. I was still insanely, head-over-heels in love with Daniel, but it was becoming obvious that his feelings were no longer reciprocated.

The change was subtle in the beginning. Where we could normally consume an entire day together, Daniel was finding ways to mysteriously vanish. Long before social media check-ins, Snapchat stories, or smartphones (you were lucky if you had a Motorola StarTac that would send and receive SMS with one hundred and forty characters or less) it was easy to go off the grid, and Daniel did—often.

Trips to the museum, followed by a walk through Central Park (to journal our feelings) that led to an afternoon movie, and finally a vegan dinner on the Upper West Side morphed into a rushed meeting at Starbucks on the way to or from somethingONE else.

I turned into Stalker Barbie, skipping acting classes and auditions to catch Daniel on another date; alas *Ken* covered his tracks and I couldn't prove anything. All that I gained was five pounds of weight because I stopped going to the gym or attending dance classes.

Six months after our show closed at Radio City, Daniel came to me and told me that he auditioned for a touring show to be a backup dancer for a Christian music singer—and he booked the job. He was leaving the following day and would be gone for six weeks. Upon hearing the news I thought my head would explode. I was one step away from having a Mariah Carey meltdown (the first one in Times Square circa TRL).

Part VI: Life After Love

With the absence of Daniel, my social life was getting back on track. It was the first time since coming out that I wasn't joined at the hip, so I might as well take advantage of the situation. Although I didn't have many gay friends, I had a small group of friends who were more than ready to support my gay lifestyle. Tracie, a choreographer and dance teacher, was my closest confidant. She was the artistic director of her own company that I occasionally danced for, and while we were nearly the same age, she always seemed to have more wisdom and strength.

Then there were my married friends, Matthew and Mari Beth. I met Matthew while working at Pottery Barn on the Upper West Side. (That entire experience deserves its own book. In the meantime, I'll elaborate more on that story in *Faced With Fame*.)

Matthew was my manager at work and my only male role model by day. Matthew was enrolled in culinary school, a chef in training, avid soccer lover, style conscious, and the cattiest straight guy I'd ever met. He was the perfect dude for me.

His wife, Mari Beth was there to be the voice of reason and keep the two of us in check—she was also the master of delivering a dry one-liner that would have us laughing through brunch. These three became my sanity during a time when doctors might have labeled me manic.

The first letter from Daniel came two weeks into his baptismal tour. It was a lengthy description of his cast, focusing primarily on the males. No surprise there. The shock came when he casually mentioned that he and his fellow ensemble members had decided to take a vow of abstinence upon the council of their Born-Again-Christian-Pop-Rock Leader.

Tracie decided that I needed to stop long distance pseudo-dating a "new age head case who bailed town to go on a Christian Cool-Aid crusade", and get out into the New York gay scene before I passed my prime. I reminded Tracie that I was 22 and she reminded me that I was practically a grandpa in Gayland. That's why I love Tracie—she never held back. She had a point. I'd been out of the closet in New York for nearly eight months and although I'd undergone a sparkling costume change (thanks, mom!) I hadn't yet had my Gaytillion.

We'd start each night at Vintage on 9th Avenue. It was equal distance between the two most approachable gay bars at the time: Posh and the more trendy Barrage. The latter was one building away from my apartment, which made it much easier to stumble home after drunken make-out sessions with random guys who weren't Daniel.

Tracie and I found great joy in challenging one another to act outside of our comfort zone. Three dirty Martinis into our evening, and she would dare me to walk up to complete strangers (whom I found HOT) and start a conversation. I had no clue what to say or expect, but generally it worked in my favor.

For example, Juan, the Nautica model, who was so gorgeous I nearly had an orgasm just staring into his green eyes. I didn't think

I stood a chance with Juan; fortunately Juan was into short funny dudes who were comfortable with teenage make out sessions in public places.

Then there was *another* Juan, the construction worker from Puerto Rico who "accidentally" stumbled into a gay bar. The rub-and-tug that ensued in the bathroom later was definitely intentional. I felt a little dirty (especially considering that Tracie had a bird's–eye view of my scandalous behavior) but because of her supportive nudge to explore my sexuality, I thought JUANot?

Hung over and feeling sleazy, I would recap my wild nights out with Tracie over brunch with Matthew and Mari Beth. The first few weeks I could tell that Mattie and MB (or M&M as I affectionately referred to them) did not believe my stories. By the first month of my new club-kid lifestyle, their saucer-eyes had narrowed and they couldn't get enough of my tea.

Daniel's letters came few and far between, each more bizarre and cryptic than the last. The most recent one informed me that his tour would be ending at Madison Square Garden and Daniel had left a ticket in my name at Will Call. I was confused. Were there really that many Born Again Christian Rock lovers living in Manhattan? Also, why wasn't I more elated about Daniel's return?

I arrived at the theater early, and it's a good thing I did. Incredibly, the concert was sold out—Christ was winning, even in New York City. I picked up my ticket and found my place near the stage.

The concert was a parody flashback to my days in Catholic CCD classes. Instead of hearing Miss Defori proclaim the good word of Jesus, I witnessed a live three-hour resurrection. What Christian Rock concert would be complete without dancers wearing costumes bedazzled with Crucifixions, twirling around flaming pyrotechnics?

It was an awakening for me all right; I realized Daniel had followed the flock back into the closet.

Afterward, I met Daniel at his tour bus. Despite the cult-like content of the concert, his performance was stellar. I was happy to see his face. Regrettably, I was greeted with a handshake instead of a hug. He took me on a quick tour of the bus, introduced me to the other male dancers, and showed me where they slept. I was surprised to see four tightly stacked cubbyholes. I asked, "Who sleeps on top?" The joke was not well received. I guess after six weeks of pent-up celibacy, no one was going to acknowledge the elephant in the room. After an awkward pause, we joined the rest of his cast for dinner sans drinks; apparently Jesus had changed his mind about wine.

The following morning I reached out to Daniel to see if he was able to meet for a proper reunion. I could hear the uncertainty in his voice, but I decided to be bold and demand his time.

I was the first to arrive at Zen Palate, and requested a table that would allow for some privacy. He appeared shortly after and this time he greeted me with a warm embrace. He was excited to share his journey with me, and while I wasn't especially interested in his newfound following, I was intrigued to hear how he had managed to resist temptation. Four minutes into our *date*, I realized Daniel had changed. Similar to when Madonna started speaking with a British accent, something was different, but as far as I could tell it was not for the better. What caught me off guard was how much I had grown, too. I still found him physically irresistible, but it was dawning on me that Daniel was not the confident, enlightened man that I had designed him to be in my mind.

After dinner I offered to walk Daniel home. I was still fishing for answers and his lake was murky. Never afraid to dive head first into confrontation, I asked him point blank if he was going back into the closet.

His face turned porcelain white and he stopped in his tracks. He was not ready for me to initiate such a direct dialogue. At that moment, he realized that he wasn't the only one who had changed. I had become much more secure in my ability to articulate my thoughts and unapologetic about asking for clarification.

By the time we reached the revolving glass doors of his building he had confessed his uncertainty about coming out. At one point, as seriously as Sally Field delivers her monologues in *Steel Magnolias*, he asked me if I would run off and join a monastery with him. "MONKcuse me?" I was flabbergasted. On the one hand, I was still enough in love with him that for a split second I actually imagined in my mind what that might be like. Until I contemplated the vow of celibacy—with which Daniel had had a six week head start. I asked if we would be able to have sex before we robed up, and he shot me a look of disapproval—he was already turning on the Catholic guilt.

I woke up the next morning with that uncomfortable lump in my throat that I hadn't experienced since coming out. I replayed the conversation in my mind like it was a GIF on Tumblr.

The next time we got together it was like he had amnesia. He never mentioned the monk nonsense again. We started to get back on track with our life before he left on the Christian dance crusade. Our sexual activity, which had suffered during the first few weeks of his return, had found a new climax—literally. He might not have been hooking up with Holy-hunks on the road, but our playtime in the bedroom was Born-Again.

After a particularly sticky New York evening, Daniel decided to get something off his chest. He was quiet for a few minutes as we laid in his tiny room listening to the sound of his air conditioner muffle the roar of summer on the Upper West Side. Drained and emotional, I knew that whatever he was holding in was going to be more explosive than what had erupted moments before.

Sure enough, the silence was broken with a match strike that would ignite a forty-minute firework display along Central Park West.

"I'm moving back to Canada—I've thought about this for a long time, and there is no talking me out of it. I hope that you'll come visit me often."

Nuclear rage was instant. Without pausing for a breath, I launched into a destructive Russell Crowe rant. I concluded that he really was going back into the closet.

He'd already confided in me that his family would never accept his lifestyle as a gay man, and suddenly, the war was over. The only thing that remained in the rubble was my sympathy for him.

I was fortunate to have a family who would love and accept me even if they didn't understand my struggle. More to the point, I was strong enough to love myself and face who I really was, whether I had the support of my family and friends or not. Daniel played the part of a strong, enlightened, artistic, well-educated, and confident man—but even after all of those self-help books and intellectual conversations in trendy tea rooms, he was weak and terrified to accept his true potential.

His one-way ticket to Canada was purchased, giving himself only three days to pack up and say his goodbyes. I was pissed that I had to share the last three days with his other friends, but rather than fighting it, I decided I would enjoy what was left of my life with Daniel in New York.

I stared out of the window of a Lincoln Town Car as we drove across the midtown bridge. I was fantasizing how this moment would play out in a Hollywood movie (if Hollywood actually made movies with gay people portraying anything other than clichés). I imagined that I would convince Daniel's character to pull over in the middle of New York rush hour traffic and walk to the edge of the bridge. We would profess our unending love for one another, embrace with a passionate kiss, and throw ourselves over, plunging to our deaths into the dirty and frigid East River. Not exactly a romantic comedy, but it's where my head was. Let's face it, Hollywood can always use a reboot of a timeless classic with a gay spin.

We exchanged our goodbyes on the curb in front of Air Canada; I studied his face, I inhaled his scent, I grasped at his hand until he pulled away—my instinct knew what my heart wasn't ready to accept yet. It was the last time I ever saw Daniel.

I received a letter three months after Daniel's retreat to Canada. I studied the four pages of unnecessarily obscure vocabulary words and stream-of-thought ramblings, to uncover that he was telling me not to visit him—ever.

I shared the letter with my brunch crew and they all had the same thought: "what straight man writes a four page letter to another man in calligraphy?" We all had a good laugh as we tossed back our third round of mimosas and I flirted with our server/actor. (I left with his number).

Epilogue

No matter how many years have passed I still think about Daniel from time to time and wonder if he was ever able to work through his demons. Is he happy? Is he out? Does he realize how deeply he scarred me?

In any case, I owe a tremendous amount of my happiness, success, and personal wellbeing to him. I always believed that one day I might reach the destination of unconditional acceptance, but I got lost in the fear along the path. Daniel was my escape route. With every step that he took back into the closet, I confidently marched further out. He made it safe for me to expose my darkest truth and start living an honest life. The weight of the world had been lifted off my shoulders and there was no way I was going to carry that distortion ever again. No career or person—or hot man in a pair of Calvin Kleins—is worth betraying my inner being for.

Showmance

Radio City Music Hall is the home of the "World Famous Radio City Rockettes", a bunker of livestock beneath the stage, and a bunch of *theater people* crammed into dressing rooms backstage. It was natural in this setting that hay—and hormones—went flying through the air.

Rivaling *Sex and the City* with an impressive amount of alcohol and multiple breakdowns during a year's worth of brunches with friends, I finally moved on from the Canadian coward who went back into the closet. I spent the next year playing the New York City *meat-and-greet* in the gay community and quickly discovered that I was not a whore. If the gay world had someone as promiscuous as Charlie Sheen, I would be the opposite of him.

I enjoyed the casual flirtation and banter of a first date but soon discovered that most gay men, even those who proclaimed they were looking for a relationship, really just wanted to get off—and then onto the next.

After an assemblage of bad dates that included: a lawyer who was "into" me until he discovered that I was an actor and then dumped me in the middle of dinner (I paid for the check); an adorable performer who was busy *performing* with five other guys, while courting me (I paid for the tests); and the aspiring writer who invited me to lavish dinners and jazz concerts (I paid for the tickets), I decided that I would refocus my energy on my budding acting career.

I divided my time between booking parts on soap operas, learning lines, working out at the gym, expanding my craft in acting classes, and flirting with unavailable straight men in Starbucks. I had too much free time on my hands—and very little money in the bank—so when the first day of rehearsal finally arrived, I was ready.

I approached the 51st street stage entrance to Radio City Music Hall with my game face on. I was an old pro confronting the rehearsal process for my third season of the Christmas Spectacular. I had victoriously survived two previous seasons on the stage, which was not an easy task considering the delicate balance of corporate communication and artistic egos. Only two years earlier I endured coming out on the majestic stage, creating a bonus scene for the cast and a lucky audience of six thousand, giving me the sense of confidence that I could conquer anything.

Midway through the first day of rehearsal I cornered my friend, Sam, who was also in the ensemble. Sam was the Laurel to my Hardy, the Rogers to my Astaire, or most accurately the Patsy to my Edina. Notice I'm always the fat one? It's true; Sam could eat whatever he wanted and still maintain the perfect dancer's physique—bitch.

"Who's the new guy?"

"I don't know [long pause and a sly smile creeps onto Sam's face] but he's mine!"

"No Sam, I claimed him first." So much for my giving up on men declaration, which I had made only weeks before catching a glimpse of this mysterious musical theater hunk.

We continued our lighthearted exchange until we were called back into the rehearsal room, where I maintained a dedicated and watchful eye on my new show crush and surveillance on all of the other curious chorus boys who were drooling in the wings.

I was not the only one drawn to his long legs, tight butt, trim torso, golden brown hair, and strong jaw line. At our pre-opening gala the night before, my friend Melissa and I spotted John Dooooh-MY-GOD wearing an impeccably tailored charcoal grey Dolce & Gabbana suit and instantly fell in love.

Melissa is the female version of me. Confidant, opinionated, passionate, uninhibited, loyal, blatantly honest, she laughs out loud, and she uses Ranch dressing like it's a life saving elixir; on everything. She is also one of the most gorgeous women I've ever met, inside and out. Utterly unaware of how talented she truly is, but assured with blonde hair, blue eyes, and a smile that will unlock the key to almost any kingdom. Oh, and she grew up with my ex-girlfriend, Kristen, so yeah—that was tough.

Lucky for me, Melissa remained open-minded and forgiving enough to see past the drama and realize that likeminded people are hard to find in New York City. Our friendship was conceived through a mutual introduction and forged into a lifelong bond of indulging in fried foods covered in mayonnaise-based dips.

When we weren't busy stuffing our faces, we both enjoyed an adventure, and Santa's secret stud became our new mission. In an effort to gather information and cover our bases, Melissa and I recruited Sam to join our gang.

It's hard to be infatuated with someone if you can't obsessively scribble his or her name down over and over again in your journal each night before you go to bed. Our first goal was to find out his name.

We were all adults, so the natural approach would have been to introduce ourselves on the first day of rehearsal but we were too busy acting like school kids and we missed that opportunity. Now we were forced to infringe on a conversation he was having with a group of our colleagues who understood proper social protocol.

Melissa is exceptional at barging in on conversations; hence Sam and I nominated her to lead us into the flock of vultures that were nestled cozy on the floor of our green room. Favorably, we knew several of the other performers in the group from the previous season, so we were able to introduce ourselves to the man of the hour under the guise of catching up with old friends.

During our exchange a seat opened up next to the heartthrob and I pounced. I causally introduced myself and he reciprocated with a firm, self-assured, and still warm response, "I'm Jeffrey, you can call me Jeff."

Our eyes locked while we shared small talk. In the remaining moments that we had before going back into Christmas choreography mode, I learned that Jeff had just moved to New York City from Los Angeles. He was well spoken, undoubtedly kind, and respectfully restrained. It only took three sentences to realize how intelligent, passionate, and witty he was—when he lovingly mentioned his mother, I recognized that his family was more important to him than anything else. At once, I knew this was the man I was going to spend the rest of my life with.

My only problem: I still didn't know which team he played for. Jeff was charming and coy with seemingly everyone he talked to during rehearsals. His appearance was what you'd expect from a wasp, but could very easily be mistaken for a man who enjoys the company of other men. He was a gentleman, with a hint of edge to him. He mixed classic patterns with clothes that you might see on the runways or in high-end department stores and think, "Who in the world would wear that?" Then you'd see it on Jeff and think, "Wow, he's got style and not afraid to show it."

Like a montage from *The Devil Wears Prada*, each day, Jeff would walk into the rehearsal hall wearing a new outfit; dress slacks with a well paired T-shirt, Diesel jeans and a polo shirt, a cashmere turtleneck with designer track pants—and my personal favorite—tie-dyed corduroy pants with an Armani tux shirt and Prada sneakers.

By our second week of rehearsal, I was head over heels for Jeff. He had no clue and every day new cast members were unabashedly throwing themselves at him. It was time to amp up my game, but my track record in the New York dating market was nowhere near a qualifying Olympic time.

My present came on the Eighth day of Christmas—rehearsal. We had just finished running a musical number from the show in which the entire cast is dressed like Santa. It's a jolly number with a fun tap dancing break. Just because Santa is heavy doesn't mean he's not a hoofer. It was my favorite scene in the show and it was noticeable because our director asked me to demonstrate the opening choreography to our entire cast in order to help conjure the spirit of St. Nick.

Following my riveting performance our stage manager called a ten-minute break. Thank god! I had to pee. As I was walking toward the bathrooms, Jeff stopped me and said, "You did a really wonderful job with that."

"Thanks," I said quickly and then hurried off to the bathroom.

My heart was racing and my stomach was tingling in that funny kind of way, some of which dissipated after I relieved my bladder, but a euphoric throbbing replaced the liquid lost. I splashed water on my face and, after checking the stalls to make sure I was alone, I had a conversation with myself in the mirror. "This is your chance. He complimented you—go for it. Otherwise that annoying dance captain is going to weasel his way into Jeff's arms before you do!"

I turned left out of the bathroom and found Sam and Melissa huddled in the usual corner. After reenacting what had just happened I informed them that we needed to plan a group outing. This way I could casually ask Jeff out on a date, without it actually being a date. (Because that's what you do when you're a seventh grade girl with a crush—or me.)

I should mention that when Jeff shares *his* version of this story, he claims that I was a cocky jerk who brushed him off when he gave me the compliment. In truth, I was so nervous that I peed my pants a little bit and had to run away before I threw up in his face—bodily fluids from one area at a time please. As a rule, people don't intimidate me. But Jeff wasn't *people*. He was a Christmas miracle and I was overwhelmed by his divinity.

After rehearsal that day I summoned the courage to confront him. It had been a long week, and I remembered how overwhelming all of the material can be the first year, so I offered to help him if he needed to review anything.

He seemed caught off guard but very grateful of my offer, which reminded me that he was only human. From that point on, our conversation was relaxed and playful. I casually mentioned that a few of us were meeting at the 42nd street AMC to catch *The Truth About Charlie* featuring the hot underwear-model-turned-rapper-turned-actor, Marky Mark Wahlberg. His face lit up as he said, "How can I refuse those abs?" GAYm on! In one fabulous exchange he confirmed that he was playing on my team; and did he just agree to a (group) date with me?

We reconvened at the theater later that evening and after loading up on popcorn, candy, and soda we made our way into the mega movie stadium where I had strategically pre assigned seats to everyone in the group (before Jeff arrived) to ensure that I had the spot next to his.

The truth about the movie is that it was slow and there weren't enough nude scenes with Marky Mark to make up for it. Melissa and I had lost interest in the film and started to dish about Jeff. He was seated to my right and had occasionally tangled his fingers with mine on our shared armrest. She had just counseled me on my next move when I felt Jeff's elbow jab me in my side.

"I'm sorry, are we being too loud?"

"No, look—he's about to get naked." Jeff proclaimed while pointing at the screen.

As my eyes readjusted to the enormous chiseled abs, rock hard pectorals, and python arms of Mr. Calvin Klein on the screen ahead, my heart sank with the anguish; Jeff is out of my league. He wants a man with the body of a Greek God and I'm just a chorus boy with the body of Bart Simpson.

Stimulating images of toned flesh flashed across the screen, while I sat in darkness pretending to watch the remainder of the movie. My mind struggled to find a convincing argument as to why Jeff might decide that I'm the man-boy for him.

Afterwards the group went for a nightcap, because when you're in your twenties in New York City everything begins and ends with alcohol. We relocated to a popular Hell's Kitchen bar that catered to *theater* people like ourselves--broke but fabulous—and we found a cramped table in the trendy, loud, and cheap spot.

Again, I found a way to wedge myself next to Jeff and in an effort to save myself another heartache; I cut right to the chase.

Me: "That was a fun movie."

Jeff: "Yes, I think we all saw the twist at the end, but (very flirty towards me) we got to see Mark Wahlberg naked."

Me: "Uh, hum. Uh, hum. That was nice. So what's your type?"

Jeff: "My type? I don't really have a type. I'm interested in all kinds of people."

Me: "That's so wonderful." (Almost too excited.)

His authentic response settled my nerves and the conversation evolved into a straightforward and friendly exchange about love, our future goals, and our families. Unlike every other man in Manhattan, Jeff's agenda was clearly to find a soul mate and not a sex toy.

Our friendship intensified in the days following our first (group) date. Because of our demanding show schedule we almost never had a day off so we made the most of our time in between shows backstage laughing, reading, writing, playing games, eating, and dreaming about our lofty futures. When we weren't at the theater, we were enjoying dinners out, attending events, going to movies, and journaling together. We started a gay relationship at lesbian speed.

Jeff validated my first impression of him during a steamy make out session back at his well-situated apartment near Central Park South. Several weeks into our relationship, I attempted to direct our R-Rated sex scene into a scandalous NC 17. He politely redirected the shot, explaining—like a true gentleman—that he really wanted a future with me and suggested that we continue to get to know each other on a deeper level before we confuse things with sex.

Had I crossed the line? I pulled Sam aside in the dressing room the following day and divulged what had happened. Sam did his best to hide his reaction, but the Wendy Williams "Girl, you got a problem!" look was evident. There was only one thing I could do. I sent Sam over to appraise Jeff's emotional mood.

Moments later Sam returned to our dressing table with an even more concerning look on his face. I recognized this smirk as the "I have dirt on you and if you ever cross me I will release it to the universe" look. Examples of this expression can be observed regularly at gay clubs across the country and at dinner parties throughout Washington D.C.

Sam twirled into the seat and recounted Jeff's words with a twinkle in his eyes.

"Sam, I don't kiss and tell. Please inform Matthew, that if he wants to know how I feel, he should come over and talk to me directly."

Gulp. What? Jeff is breaking gay protocol. Even a freshman gay man understands the benefit of the GBF (gay best friend) who acts as a mediator between potential lovers, giving everyone involved a safe space to express their feelings without the embracement of face to face rejection. They are also the first to tell you when you're getting fat.

Never one to leave things lingering too long out of fear of certain poaching—especially in a men's chorus dressing room—I swallowed my ego and mustered up my confidence. By the time I'd reached Jeff he was waiting for me with an enormous grin on his face.

"Sam told me that you wanted to see me?"

"Is that all he told you?" Jeff asked in a sly and sassy manner.

"No. He said that..." I repeated the words that Sam was told to quote verbatim back to Jeff.

Laughing, Jeff pulled me down to the foam mattress that he would rest on between shows and cuddled me next to him. He informed me that he didn't believe in locker gossip—any gossip—for that matter and that I should always feel comfortable directing all of my questions or concerns towards him. "It's part of building trust and intimacy."

With every shared conversation, intimate moment, and emotional encounter I was falling deeper in love with Jeff. I had been down this path before, literally: Daniel and I took the same route from our dressing rooms to the stage every day exchanging familiar sentiments. Only with Jeff, I understood our attraction and respect for each other was mutual.

The word "showmance" is often used in the industry to define a relationship that blossoms when two performers working on a project hook up. Famous examples are endless.

There are the obvious; Brad and Angelina, Tom and Nicole, and Robert Pattinson and Kristen Stewart.

There are the classics like Goldie Hawn and Kurt Russell, Susan Sarandon and Tim Robbins, and Brad and Gwyneth.

Finally, there are the "publicity" showmances like Ben Affleck and JLo, Ben Affleck and Jennifer Garner, Tom Cruise and [fill in the blank]. These people were undoubtedly forced into a showmance by their manager, the movie studio, or a publicist to demonstrate their lust for one another in order to convince the general viewing audience to accept their noteworthy lack of chemistry—or in Garner's case, to climb the Hollywood hunk ladder.

Our relationship continued to flourish and our conversations shifted from philosophical projections to more concrete plans. Christmas Eve was upon us, and Jeff had invited me to join him in New Jersey to meet his father's side of the family. As we drove through the winding roads that led to a picturesque snow covered house, my stomach started to twist. I was nervous, but I did my best to hide my apprehension with a big smile.

Before we could get through the rustic threshold, a swarm of relatives, including Jeff's father, surrounded us with smiles, hugs, and hot apple cider. I was introduced to everyone and within minutes I was playing games with his nieces and nephews, learning about Jeff's childhood from his aunt, and bonding with Jeff's father, Earle. The highlight of the evening was when Jeff's cousin gathered everyone around the VCR and popped in a video; we all sang Christmas carols while watching a log burn on a TV set. It was a real Hallmark channel moment.

The next afternoon, Christmas Day, I'm sitting cozy next to Jeff at our cast dinner. All of our friends were enjoying a catered feast with loads of the traditional trimmings, and as I got up to get more stuffing (of course), I asked Jeff if he wanted anything. Upon his response, "No thank you," I said, "Sure. Love you."

Wait, what!? Did I really just say that aloud in a large rehearsal room that had been temporarily converted into a makeshift dining room to feed 36 Rockettes, 30 ensemble performers, 6 little people, Mr. and Mrs. Claus, Bambi (the head animal wrangler), 5 of her camel-dung covered crew, and 20 members of IATSE (the tough NY stagehands union)?

Sam and Melissa looked up as Jeff grabbed my arm before I could dive into the chocolate cake and eat around my feelings.

"What did you just say?" Jeff asked in an intense, unreadable tone.

"Nothing," I attempted in a very uncasual voice.

"No, I'm pretty sure you said something." He started to tease a bit.

"I said—I love you." My face was now so red that I could see the Rudolph hue bounce off of my cheeks.

"I love you, too," he said while making eye contact with me and then sharing the acknowledgment with the rest of the room.

It was a startling juxtaposition to the last romantic encounter I had at Radio City Music Hall. Instead of being annihilated for expressing my feelings, I had been publicly accepted—no—loved.

Later Christmas Day, we exchanged fancy presents. I bought Jeff a Louis Vuitton wallet and he gave me a Tiffany & Co. keychain complete with a key to his apartment.

We're both men who enjoy material goodies but it was the gift of *love* that sealed our fate that Christmas.

As our show was nearing the end of its run we decided to have "the talk." Every performer who's ever become romantically involved with a co-star experiences a moment when the two must decide if their showmance has the endurance to sustain a third act, or if it's time to bring down the curtain and exit the stage in separate directions.

Unequivocally, sacrifice-my-kidney, in love, I knew that I was ready to grow old with Jeff by my side. Building our careers, traveling the world, laughing at one another's annoying habits, raising a family, and (maybe) getting fat together.

But did he feel the same? His answer was a swift and uncomplicated, "Yes."

Faced With Fame

Life was anything but glamorous for me as a twenty-one-year-old closeted chorus boy working at the Pottery Barn in New York's art-endowed and trendy Lincoln Center area on the Upper West Side. In between fluffing pillows and the egos of Pottery Barn's rich (mostly female) clients, I spent my time working with the design team. I had exceeded the daily expected work performance of a Xennial employee and was bestowed the opportunity to carry out the aesthetic changes in the store, which were handed down through the corporate team of designers. In non-closeted-gay terms: I helped Dwain—the very confrontational and cliché gay design manager—arrange seasonal displays, false-front candles, rearrange well-manufactured slipcover sofas, and (because I was a Boy Scout and thus automatically understand how to operate a power tool) complete any project that involved a drill. All of this came with a hefty twenty-five cent an hour raise and the bonus of starting my workday at six o'clock in the morning. On the bright side, it meant working for three hours without customers!

I spent the majority of my six-month stint at Pottery Barn hating life. Dealing with affluent and utterly incompetent costumers who would return lamps they thought were broken when the light bulb simply needed to be changed. Bringing back cases of wine glasses that were obviously used for a special occasion, which the woman denied while making direct eye contact through the wine-stained and lipstick covered rim. Or my personal favorite: the angry East Side widow who returned an 8 x 10 wool rug which she "schlepped all the way from the East Side" because she didn't like the color. I didn't like the fact that it was covered in cat urine. When I mentioned this to her she insisted that it wasn't like that when she rolled it up. I suppose the huge Crate & Barrel logo wasn't there either, never-the-less Pottery Barn happily accepted the return and she walked out with the cash.

Every day was a new adventure in discovering just how shitty wealthy, superficial people in search of love, attention, or power via a retail home makeover can be. I realized quickly that my only chance of survival was to pretend that I was in a movie and everyone who entered the store was just a performer in my scene. It started out subtle. I'd arrive on "set", punch in for my "scene" and get into character. I was *Bitchy Gay Employee Number One*. The store manager was my director, my colleagues were cast mates, the annoying customers were co-stars, and everybody else was just background. Pottery Barn became my own Central Perk (a *Friends* reference for anyone living under a rock). If I were unhappy with the "direction" or an exchange with a "co-star", I would walk away from the action, rewrite my script, and start a new scene. I got so good in my "role" that I continued to live my life in New York as if I were a movie star always on camera (before reality TV) and nothing I said or did had repercussions.

In my newfound creative frame of mind, my outlook at work was positive—albeit delusional—and it was much easier to exchange a "broken" alarm clock from a crabby customer who was successful enough to own a condo in the most exclusive building across the street, but not bright enough to replace the batteries in the aforementioned alarm clock.

The confusion came when an actual famous person would enter *my* scene as a guest star.

Like the time that I was walking out of the stock room full of rage and an armful of Pottery Barn classic bath towels when just around the corner Dianne Wiest (oh my god, I LOVE Dianne Wiest) stood arguing with her daughter about an unfinished school project, while tearing through the four-hundred thread count cotton sheets without regard that I had just restocked them. I wanted to be furious at the monster that would do such a thing, but it's Dianne Wiest, so instead I offered my services and politely nodded when she explained that she's in the midst of a breakthrough with her daughter. "Don't speak." *

---

* If you don't immediately get that reference, please put your Woody Allen *issues* aside and watch *Bullets Over Broadway!* Dianne Wiest is brilliant.

During a particularly busy day when the holiday season turns average shoppers into evil elves in search of markdowns, I was working behind the cash register—a position I was not accustomed to, but occasionally forced into during high volume hours. I was far superior on the showroom floor persuading people to spend their money rather than hidden behind a machine counting back their change.

Until you've endured a mob of angry ants pushing their way through a maze of markdowns and lines that rival those of the TSA security cue at LAX, you'll never understand how horrendous the holidays are in a New York City retail shop.

"Next. *Next*. NEXT!" I would bark without looking up from the register. One at a time agitated customers would stand in front of me complaining about how long they had to wait in line, or demanding an extra discount because of the "unacceptable" delays.

"Happy Black Friday!" I would shout with a note of sarcasm, never once making eye contact, and always in character, in this instance as "Super Catty Queer Retail Snob."

"Next!"

A soft, sweet, recognizable voice politely asked, "Is there any chance I can have this gift wrapped? It's for my brother and I want him to feel special."

I sluggishly lifted my head up to make direct contact with the innocent request "I'm sorry we don't gift..." As my eyes locked on hers, I dropped to the floor behind the register and look directly to my left where my best friend and assistant manager, also named Matthew, stood looking down on me like I'd lost my marbles.

I mouthed to Matthew from under the counter, "It's Gretchen Mol! Greeeeeetchen [dramatic pause] Mol!"

Matthew calmly walked over to Gretchen, "I'm sorry, it's his first time being rude to a celebrity. I'll happily gift wrap that for your brother."

I'm sure that Gretchen's ego appreciated my reaction.

At the pinnacle of *The Rosie O'Donnell Show*'s popularity (after ignoring my store manager and reaching out to our corporate office) I was victorious in securing Rosie O'Donnell a Pottery Barn Basic Slipcover armchair directly from our store, rather than having her wait the typical three months for delivery. Rosie was very connected in the Broadway world—so when she asked me to personally deliver her chair—I considered it an exclusive invitation into the New York City theater community. After receiving the approval from our district manager I arranged to have our stock guy, Tito, join me in transporting the chair to Ro's penthouse apartment, conveniently located on the 33rd floor of our coveted uptown building.

A quick glance at our driver's licenses and a thorough examination of the luxury armchair, and we're cleared by the building's security detail. The doorman ushered us into a freight elevator, swiped his keycard, and sent us on our way. We stepped off the elevator and arrived at the penthouse door and rang the bell. To my delight, Rosie answered the door and quickly offered us a beer, which we politely declined, she shrugged her shoulders and led us into her expansive yet comfortable apartment and pointed to the exact spot she wanted the chair.

I was enamored with Rosie and never missed her show, now I'm in her apartment helping her decorate? Not even in my wildest mind-manufactured movie moment did I think something like this would really happen.

Without fuss, we positioned the chair in a radiant corner of her apartment that faced the enormous flat-screen television set, while still allowing a spectacular view of the Hudson River that *almost* compared to the high definition images on the screen.

"What an incredible view!" I stated the obvious in an effort to prolong this 'pinch me' moment.

"The river or the TV?" Ro chuckled.

"Both," I asserted.

"Yeah, we're pretty lucky. What do you do, aside from delivering furniture to annoying TV Hosts?"

I liked her style; she was deflecting the attention from her success and offered me an opportunity to shine.

I launched into a ten-minute pitch highlighting my obsession with her show and everything musical theater related, followed with a passionate declaration that I would one day be on Broadway. She reacted with her face first, exposing a look that conveyed hope and fear—then offered, "It's a tough business and you have to work hard, but I believe in you kid."

Breaking the awkward tensions, Tito interjected, "I lift weights."

Rosie responded by patting Tito on the back while simultaneously motioning us towards the door. She walked us out, but not before handing us each a generous tip.

My time at Pottery Barn ended soon after my encounter with the renowned comedian-turned-talk-show-host. Rosie unknowingly motivated me to rediscover why I'd moved to New York City. I can assure you that it was not to be verbally assaulted on an hourly basis, while returning a used duvet cover that had served as a drop cloth for a child's finger-painting lessons.

For several months I forced myself to double-up on my vocal and acting classes and I stood in line for every audition—even if they conflicted with work or it meant sacrificing my whole day to be considered—until finally I booked my first big break in the ensemble of a musical. After that, it was so long slipcovers, hello stage doors.

For a year, I consistently booked jobs and increased my visibility on the NYC theater scene. An established choreographer, whom I took classes from regularly, asked me to dance in the opening number of a Broadway benefit he was choreographing, of which the star of the number would be none other than Rosie O'Donnell.

To my dismay, Rosie was absent for the weeklong rehearsal process, and instead sent her male stand-in to learn the music and choreography. It was freakish how much he looked and acted like Rosie—for anyone who hadn't been to her house—it might have been hard to distinguish one from the other.

We made the switch from our rehearsal studio in midtown Manhattan to the New Amsterdam Theater on Broadway on a Friday afternoon. I couldn't wait to reconnect with Ro.

The cast sat in a huddle stage left exchanging gossip and swapping sexual escapades—as dancers do—while I was lurking in the upstage wing. I stalked Rosie, who was deep in conversation with her (then) wife, Kelly. I was plotting my entrance into their obviously private party of two.

The opportunity to pounce came when our stage manager called a fifteen-minute break. I bolted across the stage like Simone Biles tumbles across the floor during a routine at the Olympics. Full of adrenaline I arrived at the Queen of Daytime's feet.

"Hi Rosie, I'm not sure if you remember me—"

"You're in the musical *Chicago!*" She cut me off excitedly.

"No, but that's so funny, because that's exactly what you thought the first time we met at Pottery Barn," I reminded her.

"Oh yeah, you're the guy who sold me my armchair! It's still in the same spot, but it looks like you're not."

My "full circle moment" wasn't as vibrant as I dreamed it would be. She was polite, but I could tell that she was in no mood to make small talk. As I continued to vomit my appreciation for her encouragement, while boasting about how I'd followed through with my mission to conquer Broadway, it dawned on me: Rosie is just here to do her job. Now *I'm* the annoying co-star in her personal movie. With that realization, I excused myself and rejoined the other chorus members. Famous or not, no one wants an interloper ruining their scene.

After years of pounding the pavement in New York, I moved back to Los Angeles to continue building on my career as an actor. In Hollywood my encounters with the rich and famous doubled exponentially. The very fake movie scenes in my mind were now transpiring in very real drug stores, parking garages, and occasionally (thankfully) on working soundstages, too.

One time in the Beverly Center parking structure I shouted, "I love your work!" to Judy Greer as she passed with a bag full of Bed, Bath, and Beyond goodies. You might not recognize her name, but you would know her face from literally everything. She's Jennifer Garner's best friend in *13 Going on 30;* she's Katherine Heigl's best friend in *27 Dresses;* she's Jennifer Aniston's best friend in *Love Happens;* and she was my best friend when I remarked on her exquisite taste in decorative pillows.

While searching for discount wine at a Rite-Aid in Los Angeles I stumbled into Anna Faris, who was bending forward to take a closer look at the label on a bottle of facial moisturizer. Without hesitation I blurted out, "I think you are HILARIOUS! And—I am in *love* with your husband!"

"Thanks, so am I," she confirmed and then quickly removed herself from the aisle. She and Chris Pratt are separated now, so maybe…

At the very trendy and delicious LA eatery, Joan's on Third, I once stalked Gwen Stefani and her then husband Gavin Rossdale. I carefully studied Gwen's flawlessly applied make-up as they perused pastries and stinky cheeses. I followed them as they walked hand in hand around the display of buttery carbohydrates, salty meats, and perfectly seasoned vegetables. Occasionally Gavin would lean in and playfully kiss Gwen on the cheek. I waited until they arrived at the end of the counter to inform them that there was a group of paparazzi gathered like velociraptors outside, just waiting to snap shots as they exited the building.

It didn't dawn on me until they were leaving the café that Gwen and Gavin's *people* had probably called the tabloid hunters in order to gain press. That would explain why Gwen looked so impeccable and why Gavin appeared to be so in love. The whole time I was shadowing them—I was just another sucker in their façade—only instead of waiting to see their "evidence of love" splashed across magazines at grocery stores, I got to witness it while overpaying for the most delectably, tantalizing Chinese chicken salad you will ever find.

I had the privilege of meeting *the* Ann-Margret when my friend Elise was performing in a production of *Best Little Whore House in Texas*. Our meeting backstage was brief but unforgettable.

She extended her right hand into the palm of my right hand and then—as if shifting gears in a monster truck—she guided our hands towards my lips as she uttered, "Enchanté." She smelled like expensive perfume and a lifetime of Hollywood secrets.

Speaking of Hollywood secrets… After I had paid my dues in Los Angeles, I started to work more frequently on television. During a live production of a televised comedy variety show, I got to sing and dance with Jason Alexander, who was playful and talkative during our rehearsal process. We arrived in Las Vegas for the taping and he spent most of his time gambling. I don't know if he won or lost but he hit a jackpot on camera—and when he found out that the ensemble wasn't invited to the wrap party afterwards, he went out of his way to make sure that the producers added us to the guest list.

During that same gig, I got to rub elbows with some of my Hollywood heroes backstage in the green room. I shared appetizers with Tom Hanks and Rita Wilson, who are both as generous and charismatic off camera as they are on. I watched Steve Martin snub Faith Hill—right in front of Tim McGraw, who is unexpectedly hot. I discussed politics with Julia Louis-Dreyfus, who is confident, gorgeous, and genuine. Oh, and I stood next to Leonardo DiCaprio backstage as we watched the brilliant Wanda Sykes deliver her comedy routine. After the punch line of her final joke, Leo turned to me in full-blown laughter, locked eyes with me (they were a stunning shade of blue I didn't know existed), and squeezed my shoulder. I know that it was just an instinctual release of pure joy shared with a fellow performer, but I like to think that he really wanted to embrace me.

One of my favorite jobs ever was working on the Netflix series *Wet Hot American Summer: First Day Of Camp,* which was the prequel to the cult movie from ten years earlier. I was hired to play a camp counselor at a Jewish Day Camp who was in the ensemble of the original show, *Electro City.* It was as hysterical as it sounds.

The cast included a who's who of A-List actors, but I spent my days working with Amy Phoeler (GENIUS), Paul Rudd (FEARLESS), Michaela Watkins (LEGENDARY), John Early (SHAMELESS; in a brilliant way), and Marguritte Monroe—who somehow managed to keep a straight face and deliver a performance that was sincere and grounded.

I arrived to work early every day, not just for the delicious craft service (although the food on the shoot was an epic journey of culinary creativity), but because we would spend our mornings in the make-up and hair trailers laughing our guts out. I was surrounded by Hollywood success stories that elevated my game. They were extravagant with their time, energy, and creativity. Everyone on the set felt included in their club, which was a master class in how to hit a mark, deliver a line, improvise a scene, and still remain kind to everyone. I know that sounds like something every actor should be capable of—but trust me—there are a lot of celebrities who forget where they came from.

A decade into my dance career in Los Angeles, my body began alerting me that I was no longer twenty-something and it might be time to diversify. Despite what my fifth grade teacher Mrs. Trevor thought, my outgoing and talkative nature helped me cultivate relationships with a few industry professionals who assisted my transition into the world of choreography.

I started off choreographing small background scenes for music videos, independent films, and television. My specialty was working with talented comedic actors who had great timing with lines, but needed help with their footwork. Along the way I choreographed for: Megan Mullally (a lovely person with great rhythm and flawless skin); Henry Winkler (a Hollywood legend and a bit impatient); Armie Hammer (tall, good looking, and very quick to pick up the steps); Ben

Stiller (hard working, very collaborative, and a lot more serious than you'd expect); and my favorite. . . Rebel Wilson, who was real, witty, and willing to attack a pirouette in a pair of fabulous pumps.

But of all the stars that I've had the privilege of sharing space with, the down-to-earth *dish* I devoured during lunch with Parker Posey has stuck with me through my triumphs and tragedies.

I was sitting at a café table with Jeff toward the back of my favorite downtown NYC lunch spot (because my surrogate sister, Tara, worked there and would sneak us free food) shoving down a mouth full of pitta and hummus, when out of the corner of my eye I see Parker Posey walk through the front door.*

Knowing what a huge Parker Posey fan I am (I can quote every line she utters in *Waiting For Guffman*), Tara purposefully walked her past our table, winking at me as she sat the Darling of Indie films at the corner booth beside us.

It took me about 0.5 seconds to explain to Jeff that I was going to go into full geek mode and be *that* person who barges in on a celebrity while they're trying to eat lunch. Before he could even get the words, "Go for..." I was up and at her table.

"Excuse me, Parker, I don't want to disturb you..."

I hardly finished my sentence before Parker chimed in, "Disturb, disturb!" Coupled with a comedic and welcoming arm gesture as if she were conducting an orchestra of appreciation—classic Parker.

She invited me to sit and, in turn, I invited Jeff to join us. I noticed that she had a script in front of her. I raved about how marvelous she was and launched into a rapid-fire line of questioning that included: "What's it like to work with Christopher Guest?" "What's your favorite film that you've worked on?" "If you could play any part, what would it be?"... And most importantly, "What is *that* script?"

She offered a candid response to every question—the script was a new Christopher Guest movie called *Best In Show* (AH-mazing!)—and she shared some insight on Christopher's process for creating cult classics.

We continued to talk for another twenty minutes about the life of an actor. We discussed acting techniques, auditions, booking big parts, fame, and (the obvious) dealing with psycho super fans; her outlook

---

* Fact: I have the born ability to spot a celebrity from approximately 20 miles away.

was enlightening. I was a twenty-something actor studying theater in New York City, dreaming that I might one day get to do movies like Parker Posey. She divulged that no matter how many movies she's done or how successful she may appear to be, she's still just a person trying to get a job so that she can pay the rent on her tiny studio apartment in the West Village.

Talk about humble. I relish "light bulb moments" and Posey's revelation was the neon sign I needed to digest the simple truth. Ordinary people often fill their days fantasizing about the perks of fame to avoid reality. Celebrities spend their days pretending to be "normal" people on screen, but in reality, they long to escape the spotlight when it encumbers their personal life. In the end, we're all just trying to make sense of the script we've written for ourselves—hopefully we're kind to the co-stars in our scene along the way.

Birthday Parade

It's no wonder that I have unrealistic expectations when it comes to celebrating my birthday—not every child gets their very own birthday parade. Just like the Queen of England, I strode down Main Street while my adoring family genuflected and curtsied to my Royal Honor.

On May 4, 1980 I made my first royal appearance marching along the single lane highway wearing short brown polyester track shorts with white piping, a yellow Snoopy T-shirt, rainbow strapped flip-flops, and a sun visor. Blissfully in sync with the brass trumpets that blared from the high school band in front of me, I hoofed it down the pavement with blue and gold pom-poms shaking in my hands. I was two years old, and the taste of notoriety and praise went straight to my perfectly shaped head.

Gleaming brightly as pedestrians waved and cheered for me, I was utterly unaware of the procession of historical cars, floats presented by the Chamber of Commerce and local businesses, Shriners, and the Grand Marshall who followed behind, impatiently waiting for me to get tired and clear the path so that they could continue with the festivities of the annual Blossom Day Parade.

My birthday coincided with our town's yearly celebration ushering in the spring harvest with music, food, and craft fairs. Whether out of opportunity or frugality, my parents—with the loving support of their parents—decided that it was perfectly normal to allow me to believe that unlike any of the less worthy friends I went to school with, I was illustrious enough for the community to host a parade in my name.

To my parents' good fortune—further validating an absurd standard—my sister (two years my junior) was born on September 5, 1980, synchronizing with the fall Apple Harvest Festival. Every year, Shiree Antoinette Shaffer twirled like a princess along the very same path in her own birthday procession, which was really the Pioneer Day Parade.

Logical observation would affirm two things: One, our town orchestrated a lot of parades; and two, my parents had no problem with deception. Don't even get me started on the stupendous lengths they went to prolong the truth of Santa Claus from us. Allow me just to say that I was in sixth grade when it dawned on me that Santa's beard had the same specks of Copenhagen that my dad would often have in his moustache.

I was in third grade when my parents decided to relocate our family to Southern California. In addition to being ripped from my grandparents and my beautiful golden Cocker Spaniel, Popcorn, I was unknowingly saying farewell to my fairytale birthdays. It was unlikely that my parents could convince the city of Los Angeles to throw their eight-year-old son an annual parade. Although if my dad actually uttered those words aloud he might have heard just how *fabulous* the idea was and saved me a lot of heartache later in life.

My first birthday in Los Angeles I had no friends. I settled for a vaguely lifelike performance from three auto-tuned singing animatronic bears with tattered fur and taffeta tutus covered in sequins. While gnawing on the chemically enhanced cardboard pretending to be pizza and avoiding the seriously stained colorful carpet, I was choking on the fact that I had traded a royal birthday tradition for scores of tiny snot nosed brats in a ball bounce, sirens and ringing bells in every direction, cheap plastic prizes—and my parents' forced enthusiasm.

Most of the birthdays leading up to my thirteenth birthday were similar in their unworthiness. Year after year, my parents tried their best to recreate the magic that I once felt marching to the beat of the small town drums. Alas my batons went un-twirled.

The morning of my lucky thirteenth birthday I woke up to a huge explosion of birthday love. Not from my mom or dad, but entirely from my sister. Shiree, who was eleven at the time, had been saving and planning for weeks in order to make sure that my entrance into teenage angst was met with a worthy extravaganza.

Every afternoon while I was perfecting my pirouettes at the dance studio, my sister would walk to the party store down the street and negotiate prices on mylar balloons, streamers, confetti bombs, party favors, and a grab-bag full of from-the-heart gifts. To top it all off, the icing on the cake was me! Long before the eatable laser printer decals, she had the cake designer frost a picture of me dancing.

My sister was so thoughtful, generous, and excited to throw me a marvelous birthday party. She invested her entire savings. Unfortunately she neglected to persuade my parents to reach out to any of my friends from school.

If I were Jewish, perhaps they would have made a bigger fuss over my right of passage into manhood. I attended enough of my friends' decadent bar mitzvahs to know how important turning thirteen is. I bet my bar mitzvah would have been held at the Food Court at the Del Amo Fashion Center Mall and I would have been okay with that. Any place where I can binge on a 4000 calorie cinnamon roll, devour meat on a stick doused with MSG, and drink an orange smoothie is a worthy place to gather with friends. Turns out we had plenty of cake to split between the four of us. As a special bonus gift, my chin erupted with mountainous acne that very morning. I used the sheet cake to cover half my face in all of the photos. Happy Birthday!

To rebound from their lack of planning for my thirteenth birthday, the following year mom and dad arranged a festive outing to Olvera Street. The historical district located in downtown Los Angeles was littered with tourists browsing kiosks exploding with Latin themed tchotchkes, an abundance of mariachi bands, and scores of restaurants promising "The Best" Mexican food. My birthday falls the day before Cinco de Mayo, which is a hugely celebrated day in Southern California. There was sure to be a bounty of food, entertainment, and yes—a lively parade. I was allowed to invite five of my best friends to join us for a day of piñatas, chips and salsa, and faux switchblade knives (there was a comb in lieu of a blade).

Tragically, the week leading up to my birthday marked a dark stain on the fabric of Los Angeles. On April 29, 1992 a Los Angeles trial jury acquitted four police officers that were caught on videotape using excessive force while arresting Rodney King.

Following the announcement of the verdict, a civil unrest began to spread across the county. All Southern California schools and institutions were immediately closed and we were sent home. By that evening several innocent people were harmed including the most famous, Reginald Denny, who was pulled from his truck and beaten— the entire event was captured on live news. My dad's office was only six blocks away from Florence and Normandie where the assault took place. Thankfully, he made it home safely, where we spent the next six days while riots, looting, fires, and killings caused widespread panic throughout Los Angeles County. Mayor Tom Bradley announced a dusk-to-dawn curfew and eventually the Army National Guard was activated. There was a parade, however it was in the form of a group of brave men and women who attempted to restore peace in our city. My birthday celebration expanded into an awakening of my soul as I mourned the loss of innocent lives, thanked God for the safety of my family and friends, and realized how divided we were as people.

By my sixteenth birthday I'd given up all expectations. I was delighted when I woke up to a showering of love from my family, followed by a new boom box with detachable speakers, a CD player, and dual-tape decks. I could finally record my favorite Mariah Carey songs off KISS FM and then make a mix tape for all of my friends—is there a sixteen-year-old boy who wouldn't want radio quality recordings of Mariah Carey?

Secretly, I had hoped that my parents would by me a brand new Ford Explorer (the pre-Mercedes Benz starter car for kids), but instead I handed over my entire savings—$1000—in order to take possession of my dad's 1987 slightly dinged five-speed Ford Ranger. Proving once again how extremely thrifty my dad is. You could say that I received the best gift that year; I learned that I should never underestimate just how far my parents would go to teach me the value of a dollar.

My twenty-first birthday was a great surprise. My girlfriend, Kristen, planned a day full of activities—most of which I ruined. She arranged a spa treatment, which included a haircut, manicure, and massage. The only problem was that I had just treated myself to a haircut and mani-pedi the day before without telling her. Every straight man wants to be impeccably groomed on their twenty-first birthday, right?

Somehow she was able to stay calm and carried out the rest of her plans. She had gathered my closest friends and her hot twin brother, who flew in from St. Louis *with party favors*, into the pool house of the home where we worked as au pairs.

We danced around the pool and grilled on their outdoor Viking range until the sun set and then we headed to downtown Chicago to party at the clubs. Our first stop was a huge club called Warehouse, which was exactly what it sounds like. After paying a hefty cover charge we were inside the enormous club popping pills and fists pumping.

There were sweaty hot people laughing and dancing in every direction. I was lost in a sea of ecstasy. Literally. I had lost my friends. I searched every corner of that club to no avail, and just as the drug induced panic started to set in, I stepped outside for a fresh perspective, and I received my second surprise of the day.

My friends were huddled next to the exit door waiting for me. It turns out my GBF (gay best friend), Devert, decided that it was okay to join the "meeting in the ladies room" and they were all thrown out. When Kristen begged the bouncer to let her back in to retrieve me, he threatened to call the police. Let's just say that Chicago in the late 90s was against unisex bathrooms.

Once I moved to New York and *finally* came out of the closet, I'd given up on birthdays. After turning twenty-one, I stopped worrying about celebrating one day of the year and opted to expand my options, making every day a party.

Soon after Jeff and I started dating, we discovered that our birthdays were only two days apart. Another sign that we were meant to be together. Jeff was celebrating a milestone birthday—his thirtieth—and we were supposed to be on a lavish cruise-ship courtesy of one of Jeff's best friends, who would also be joining us. We boarded our flight from JFK in full period costume cruise wear; Jeff loves a theme. We packed enough luggage to dress for a month; Jeff loves a costume change, too.

By the time we landed and reached baggage claim at Miami airport there was pandemonium in every direction. Half jokingly I remarked, "You'd think our cruise ship sank." Moments later we approached the check in queue and learned that the luxury liner had exploded and caught fire. Needless to say, our cruise was canceled.

I debated: Is this the right time to tell Jeff that I might be cursed on my birthday? Would he stick around for a lifetime of terrible birthday calamities? Thankfully our friend, Ari, had a big imagination and deep pockets. Jeff proved he was a go-with-the-flow kind of guy and we all relaxed into vacation mode. We partied the night away in Miami and continued the parade all the way down to the Florida Keys.

Five years later and now I was the one turning thirty. Jeff and I were living in Los Angeles and a mutual friend of ours, Michael, decided to throw me a surprise birthday bash on the beach.

With the help of Jeff, for access to my email accounts, Michael reached out to every single contact in my Google address list and all of the random people on my MySpace page. Whether I worked with you ten years ago on a shitty gig or stalked you on an early version of social media, if we once dated and you cheated on me or you were a former boss who fired me because I wouldn't sleep with you—you were invited. The intentions were right, but the due diligence was shoddy.

Michael's twin brother Chris offered his prime beachfront house to host the party, which was the perfect venue for a day of sun, swimming, and barbequing. Together, Michael and Jeff emptied their bank accounts on enough food and alcohol to keep Kirstie Alley and Lindsay Lohan in addiction for years to come.

In the days leading up to my birthday, Michael planted the seeds for an elaborate scheme that he had devised in order to convince me that he would be out of town working on my birthday. Too bad for him, a week before my birthday, I'd caught a glimpse of the "secret" Evite that he'd sent out. People really should be more vigilant about signing out of their email accounts before allowing a friend to use their computer.

On the day of my birthday I woke up to a knock on our front door—(no) surprise! It was Michael with a bag full of props for the adventure that he was about to take me on. I acted like I had no clue what was going down. Jeff, who can read me like a book, knew that I had figured it out, but he played along, too. In the end, it was a splendidly sunny day at the beach featuring a procession of friends, ex-coworkers, and a random MySpace stalker who insisted that I accept his "birthday kiss" or he'd drown himself in the ocean; favorably the lifeguard was quick to his rescue.

I turned forty this year. From my now distant youth, I recall hearing adults talk about turning forty as if it were the end of their life. "Over the hill." Nothing could be further from the truth. With every passing season I unearth a more meaningful understanding and acceptance of who I am.

I spent my fortieth birthday laying on a beach next to my husband, my best friend Tracie, and her partner Bruce. Together we sipped Lava

Flows, traversed fields of lavender, soaked in spas, splashed around waterfalls, and celebrated our bodies with beachside yoga in bathing suits. Exercising half naked in public is something I would never do in my twenties when I was overcome with self-judgment.

As the years have pranced on, my expectations have evolved, too. I no longer anticipate my birthday to mark life's victories. Whether I'm soaring through the exalted Alaskan air on a helicopter expedition to dance on a glacier (thanks to my mother-in-law), or I'm sailing on the serene Pacific, sipping champagne with friends on a sunny Tuesday afternoon in the middle of December, I bring the party with me 365 days a year. When the day comes that I utter my last breath on Earth, don't mourn for me; please—throw me a parade!

All In the Family

Despite the power struggles that can plague a duo of Type A personalities, my cousin, Bryan and I got along very well growing up. Aside from the natural rivalry that exists between the first-born males in an already competitive family, we used our leadership skills to our advantage and would often divide and conquer in order to achieve the greater good for the rest of our clan.

Bryan, nine months my senior, is a taller, leaner version of me. We both have high cheekbones and big expressive eyes—mine are hazel; his are brown. I inherited a stronger nose and he got broader shoulders, I have better hair (he's now sleek on top) and he got a thin waistline. Bryan was the first grandchild on my mom's side of the family and subsequently he was looked upon as the golden kid in our tight knit crew of nine. The first to walk, the first to talk, the first to transition from the kids' table to the adult table, the first to get a perm (yes it happened, it was the 80s), the first to go off to college, and he was the first to get married.

When we were in grade school, Bryan and I would order each other's siblings around at family gatherings. Whether we were playing tag or a game of pretend, we were always the "leaders", "managers", "principals", or "bosses" as we both loved to talk and enforce rules.

We were both infatuated with *Saturday Night Live,* so in middle school, we decided to swipe my dad's Camcorder and produce our own sketch show. It made sense that we would be the "head writers" and "lead actors"; forcing our siblings to build sets, grip (wrangling all of the cords), and act in minor supporting roles.

High school hit us, and we both struggled to fit in, while following our decided passions. Mine (in case you still haven't figured it out) was performing. His was speech and debate. And of course, we were both presidents of several student body organizations.

After graduation he began college at the University of New Mexico. He came home for Christmas break during his first year of school, when I was still a senior in high school. He anxiously pulled me aside after a family dinner and confessed, "Matthew, I can't tell you how excited I am to get back to my friends; *my* life."

I was shocked that he was so eager to return to school. Bryan was the family hero. Looking back, I can see how exhausting that pressure must have been, always carrying the burden of responsibility for the next generation of our family.

During spring break the same year, Bryan invited his brother, Brad and me to visit him at his fraternity house. I was appalled at the piles of dirty dishes stacked in the sink and the aroma of man sweat and unidentified stains on the mismatched furniture. The filthy living conditions and lack of focus or drive from the "students" was second only to the underlying homoerotic behavior of the fraternity brothers. Ass spanking, naked video game playing, and late-night drunken circle jerks; and *I'm* the one that everyone is calling a fag?

Choosing a less traditional exit strategy, I accepted an apprenticeship with a world-renowned touring concert dance company based in Chicago and moved away from home the summer I graduated. The frat house may have been a turn-on, but it was not going to enhance my fast track to the A-list. As for the education, I'm confident I learned more in the four months I spent reading, perusing masters of art in museums, and honing in on historical sights while traveling through Europe, than most kids receive in four years at school.

The first four months of my life in Chicago were brutal. I thought I was ready to get out and start my life, but I spent more time crying on the phone to my family than enjoying the Windy City's notable nightlife, infamous deep-dish pizza, and vibrant museums. My days consisted of spending two hours at the gym (foreshadowing the rest of my life thanks to my love of food and unfortunate genetic setbacks), four hours of company rehearsal, a brief respite for soup at the diner across from our studio, followed by an evening full of dance classes. On the weekends I worked double shifts at a breakfast restaurant and still didn't make ends meet. Thanks again mom and dad for subsiding my "professional" career.

During his second year of college my cousin called me up and told me he was flying to Chicago for a weekend visit. I was overjoyed. Bryan's timing was perfect. I *needed* my family. I was in rehearsals during the day and I didn't have a car; I explained that he would have to find his own way from O'Hare Airport. "It's easy. You just take the el train." Leave it to an eighteen year old me to make my cousin find his way in a new city, after he'd gone out of his way to come shake me to life.

Taking the wrong train, twice, Bryan arrived at my apartment just as I was finishing with rehearsal. We only had two days to catch up and see the sights. Wasting no time, I suggested that we go to dinner at a restaurant in downtown Evanston where one of my friends worked. It had been awhile since I enjoyed anything other than a just-add-water meal, and even though we were both young and broke, Bryan had offered to take me out in exchange for showing him the nightlife.

We spent the evening shoving our faces with free carbohydrates dipped in olive oil and Parmesan cheese, while dreaming about the future and sharing our fears about life without the safety net of our families. Bryan was confident when he offered his positive support and advice, reminding me that I was a leader with a winning personality and it was very unlikely that I would fail at anything I put my mind to.

I grew up a very cocky "go getter". I had no doubt that I would achieve the goals that I set out to accomplish; yet something happened when I moved away from home. I was lost and overwhelmed with incredible guilt. I'd spent the past three months judging myself for leaving my family to follow my dreams. Themes of selfishness and remorse danced around my mind, causing me to underachieve in rehearsals. On the few occasions that I would go out with a new friend, the second I started to enjoy myself I would become ashamed that I chose following my dreams over my family. Bryan's words were precisely what I needed to hear in order to get over the self-inflicted drama and get on with the life that I had spent every waking (and sleeping) hour dreaming of.

The following afternoon before Bryan took the Purple Line, to the Red Line, to the Blue Line to O'Hare, he cornered me in my 300 square foot apartment.

The conversation started off like an unwanted Sex-Ed conversation from your grandma. "Matthew, do you ever have feelings for boys?"

"What? *No!* Where on earth is this coming from?" Denial set in; I was hysterical.

"I thought I noticed you checking out one of the waiters at the restaurant last night, and I just wanted to see if there was something there."

"Why does everyone assume that just because I'm a performer, I'm gay?" I shouted, snapping my head back and forth, while flailing my arms in the air.

"Okay, okay, I'm sorry. I just thought that you'd feel comfortable sharing things like that with me. I want you to know that I love you and I will support you no matter what. I hope that you would do the same for me," Bryan responded with brutal compassion.

"Bryan, I am not gay, and I would not hang out with anyone who is. Let's just leave it at that!"

I thanked him for coming to visit and I walked him to his train. It was silent for the entire fifteen-minute walk to the Northwestern station until 300 yards from the train stop, out of nowhere Bryan projectile vomited all over. He claimed that something he ate the night before wasn't agreeing with his stomach. He boarded the train and we didn't speak for three weeks.

Years later, I was living in New York City. I had finally found my way out of the closet and into a 200 square foot apartment with my then boyfriend, now husband, Jeff. By now, everyone in my family knew that I was gay—okay fine—they knew the moment I declared, "I'm moving to New York City to dance on Broadway", but I had officially confirmed it by belting out an original song that ended with a sustained high-C belt, "I'm GAAAAAAAAAAAAYYYYYYYYYYY!" Sometimes it is both necessary and appropriate to play up a clichéd stereotype. Just ask the creators of *Will & Grace;* both incarnations.

I was now steadily employed as a chorus dancer and my cousin Bryan had successfully finished law school and opened up his own private practice. He was establishing a noteworthy name for himself in immigration law and would often visit New York City.

Months before Jeff and I announced that we were going to move back to Los Angeles to continue our lives together as OUT movie stars, Bryan phoned asking if he could bring his family to come visit us. He booked a suit at The Plaza—because that's what people who finish law school and have a *real* job do—and flew his beautiful wife and their two adorable children to meet Jeff.

Naturally, Jeff insisted on hosting a formal brunch for six in the shoebox we called home. Jeff arranged the Dessert Rose China around the modern designer glass table and began preparing homemade lemon zest pancakes, bacon, cheesy scrambled eggs, Maui coconut coffee, and fresh squeezed orange juice with a selection of jams, plenty of butter, and authentic Maple syrup—no Mrs. Butterworth's in our household.

Like clockwork, there was a buzz on our intercom at 11 a.m. and we welcomed the gang into our Queen-sized café. There was an exchange of introductions; Jeff took the lead on conversation with his charming chatter about the China, his joy of cooking, and love of family. Jeff is also close to his cousins and had no problem making mine feel right at home.

Finished with brunch, I suggested that we walk over to 5th Avenue for some window-shopping. Bryan's wife was now Jeff's new best friend and it was the perfect way to continue the bonding session. We would also be close to their hotel, so we could drop them off once we were done with our day.

Jeff and Bryan's family were making their way into the mega-toy store FAO Schwarz (which sadly is a toy store no more) when Bryan pulled me aside, "The next time I'm in New York, I want you guys to take me to a gay bar."

I laughed at the thought of my fiscally prudent cousin, who was wearing pleated khaki pants and an Oxford button down underneath a plaid sweater-vest with an oversized peacoat, in a gay bar in trendy NYC. Playing along, I offered up, "Seriously? Okay, why?"

"I think it would be fun to see what it's like."

"It's like a straight bar, only all the guys are trying to sleep with other guys," I confirmed.

Jeff, who had snuck back to join us and overheard the conversation, was quick to support Bryan's request. "We'd love to take you, anytime! It would be fun. The dancing is the best!" We all smiled, nodded, and met up with his wife and the kids.

We dropped Bryan and his family off at The Plaza later that evening and began walking back to the West Side. As we walked along

Central Park South, we swapped memorable moments from our day, and chuckled as we landed on the intriguing request that Bryan had made. Jeff was quick to offer a non-judgmental response: "Maybe he's curious?"

"Jeff, did you see how he was dressed? No, he's not curious. He's married. He has children. He's so conservative!" Everyone on Central Park South stopped and glared at me.

Jeff calmly responded, "People are who they say they are. Maybe he's trying to tell you something."

"No, I think he just wants to take a glimpse at my wild lifestyle and report back to our family."

"Well, don't be too sure. He seemed very sincere to me."

Jeff and I had only been dating for a year when we moved across the country, which is tough on any relationship; thankfully after several months in LA we had adjusted to our new lifestyle and routine. Regrettably, we never made good on our promise to take Bryan to a New York City gay bar.

Not too long after we moved back to Los Angeles, I was startled awake by a 3 a.m. phone call. (I always panic when the telephone rings after 9 p.m. because it's never someone calling to offer you a job, money, or laughter.) Sure enough, it was my cousin Bryan, sobbing uncontrollably.

I struggled to make out many of his words, but I was certain that something terrible had happened and I was fairly sure that someone in my family had died.

"Bryan, Bryan, I can't understand what you're saying. Can you take a deep breath and just talk slowly and clearly? Are. You. O—kay?" I heard a deep breath and then...

"I can't do this anymore. I can't take the pressure. I don't know how you did it for so long."

"I can tell you're very upset, but I still don't know what you're talking about."

"Matt [incredibly long dramatic pause] I'm gay." The words fought their way out of his mouth with such a gravity that I knew instantly this was the first time he'd acknowledged this out loud to himself or anybody.

Finally, I was first at something in this family, was the initial reaction that popped into my mind; then, *I* took a deep breath and I listened. I could hear the pain and despair in his voice. I could relate to the feelings he was experiencing. I remembered the agony and magnitude of the process. I also recalled the relief of unburdening myself; the miracle of discovering that you can live a life without constantly monitoring your reactions, feelings, and freaking out about someone discovering your dark secret.

As he finished sharing I could already hear the shift in his tone and mood. Having someone to talk to reminded Bryan that life would go on; as a matter of fact, it would be a more worthwhile and fulfilling life…. Indeed, it can get better.

So many questions jumped into my head. Who else knows? Have you hooked up with a guy yet? What will you tell your children? What will you tell your wife? What will you tell your dad?! Have you been introduced to Liza Minnelli yet? The question I decided to ask first was, "How long have you known?"

His answer was very similar to mine. He'd always suspected that deep down he was hiding from the truth. He tried his best to live a *normal* life; wife—whom he was always faithful to—and kids included, until the urge could no longer be brushed off as a casual frat house attraction. What astonished me was what he revealed next.

"Do you remember that time I came to visit you in Chicago?"

"Yes, of course."

"Well, I was actually trying to come out to you then. I wanted to test the waters before I just blurted it out, so I thought if I could get you to open up about your sexuality, that I would feel safe to do so, too. I guess I was hoping that we could come out together, to our family. Maybe that would have made it easier?"

I felt my heart shrivel up like an animated clinical video they use in schools to illustrate the dangers of heart disease to smokers. That explains why he threw up all over the sidewalk on Davis Street in Chicago. He wasn't visiting to save me—he was there to save *us*— and he hadn't been able to complete his mission. There was a lot of unexpressed expectation and pressure on Bryan's part, but I had been utterly insensitive to my cousin, when he was simply trying to let me know that he loved me unconditionally and was imploring that in return.

I could never make up for what happened ten years earlier. The torment and fear that I had faced every day when I looked in the mirror was contagious. I was overflowing with self-hate and had betrayed my inner spirit because I was afraid of what my family and friends, the world, and the entertainment industry might think of me. These inner demons prevented me from accepting myself, and in turn, my cousin. Now all I could do was offer him love. I vowed to support him whenever and however he needed me. I assured him that I would have his back when he started telling people.

Recalling everything I could from my personal soap opera, I did my best to prepare him for what to expect from friends, family, and then of course the one thing I couldn't relate to—his wife and children. My breakup with Kristen was dramatic enough (and I didn't put a ring on it). What was his wife going to do? How was she going to react? Neither one of us could know the answers in that moment, but I reassured him that with time, everything would resolve itself. We may not like the outcome, but there's always a solution.

As sure as Sarah Jessica Parker forever has a job on HBO, Bryan and his wife and children eventually worked through the process. With time, love, and a lot of communication they've evolved into their very own *Modern Family*.

One year after coming out, Bryan had already lived a more exciting gay lifestyle than Jeff and I combined. Favorably for us, Bryan has included us on his journey. We've partied in the seedy nightclubs of Puerto Vallarta; checked out hot gay dads during Disney's Gay Day (in my opinion, every day is a *gay* day in the Magic Kingdom); we cheered Bryan and his brother, Brad, on as they crossed the victory line during the AIDS/LifeCycle ride; we've danced on tables during Los Angeles Pride; and played Drag Queen Bingo with our entire family at Hamburger Mary's, where my mom decided to start a discussion about lube—it was a slippery conversation.

My cousin is now a very accomplished lawyer. No doubt one day he'll become a judge, or who knows, perhaps he'll be the first openly gay President of the United States of America? Wherever we end up, you can rest assured that we will both be somewhere overachieving—if not to motivate each other, then to prove to our family that our gay genes are a perfect fit for success.

Mole Man

I spent three weeks of my sixth grade year with a Band-Aid on my face, disguising the mole that remained deeply rooted even after I declared to my entire middle school that I was having it removed over Spring Break. There wasn't enough gauze on the planet to mask the embarrassment I felt when I had to own up to the truth.

The truth is that I was born with a tiny little birthmark just above my lip on the left side of my face. Women adored this hideous "beauty" mark and would swoon over me as a small child. I wasn't conscious of this tiny flaw until the little brown speckle decided to erupt into a mini baseball mound around fifth grade.

My milk chocolate brown mole had a public coming out on the first day of sixth grade, when my funny sidekick "friend" thought it would be hilarious to announce me as Cindy Crawford when I walked into my homeroom class for the first time. The entire class exploded with laughter, and faster than JLo changes her see-through dresses at an award show, my nickname transitioned from Fat Matt to Matt the Mole Man.

I had never been so self-conscious in my life. I was ready for my next three years at Calle Mayor Middle School to be a time of new friendships, school dances, and a trip to third base.*

Instead, sixth grade marked the beginning of a five-year obsession with hating myself on the inside. Never one to give off the illusion that I was anything other than happy, cool, confident and collected, I would

---

* I didn't even know what that meant, but I knew I was supposed to.

145

encourage jokes at my expense—even rewriting a wittier punch line. They might have been laughing at me, but at least they knew who I was; an odd thing for me to care about, but I did.

Shrimp, midget, butterball, fatboy, Mattie-The-Fatty, Fat Matt, and now Mole Man—I wasn't sure I was going to be able to handle another year…

Thankfully I found the *theatre*, and spent the rest of my adolescence focused on drama, and not my horrendous birth defect. Following graduation, I packed my bags and Mr. Molie and I moved to New York, where once again the theater embraced us.

When I moved back to Los Angeles to continue building my acting career, I hit the ground running. My Type-A personality was ready to deposit a $1,000,000.00 check, accept a star on the Walk of Fame, and buy a huge mansion in the hills. Of course before all of this could happen, I needed to convince a team of agents and managers that they should represent me as their client.

I began taking meetings around town and eventually found my way into the brittle arms of Marianne Davis. As short as she was sassy, Marianne wore clothing that was twenty years too young, perfume that was forty years too wealthy, a wig that was synthetic, costume jewelry "borrowed" from a production back when she was under contract as an actress (I'm sure), and pink acrylic nails. Her goal was to come off as a polished player in the Hollywood system, but her look conjured up more of a Golden Girls Gone Wild kind of vibe.

The crucial part of the story is that while Marianne looked like a character from The Muppets, she actually had clients working on big projects in the industry. More enticing was that she was unabashed when it came to taking action and getting people into rooms.

On our second meeting at a slightly dated, but still tasty restaurant in Beverly Hills, we discussed the urgency for new headshots. Marianne had a "marvelous" guy who was shooting A-list celebrities for lifestyle and entertainment magazines. She pulled out her day planner, which looked more like a hoarders' to-do list and passed me a sticky note with the photographer's name and phone number.

I called the "photog to the stars" to set up the initial consultation and ended the call with an appointment to shoot the following week. I spent the next four days obsessing over clothing in order to find the perfect outfit that would pop, but still allow my eyes to stand out. I carefully taped down the tags in order to return them to The Gap and Banana Republic once I was done with my shoot.

The night before my shoot I had my bags packed, I'd lost the four pounds I needed to feel camera ready and I went to bed early (and without a glass of wine) to look my best. I arrived on site fifteen minutes early. Russell was just wrapping a photo shoot with Justina Machado from *Six Feet Under*, and at that moment, I knew Marianne was legit.

Russell had an array of backdrops and props set up with a high-energy soundtrack playing, which made it easy to change clothes and transition from scene to scene. The entire time I was acting as if I was already a household name on the cover of magazines—less *People* more *GQ*. Russell seemed enthusiastic about the photos he captured, and with over five hundred frames and six costume changes, I felt confident, too.

I received the link to the online proof sheet two days later and started clicking through the thumbnails, sorting out the ones that popped from the ones that flopped. Once I gathered the perfect selection for my capricious manager—deleting any trace of the eyes-half-opened, mouth-half-crooked, gut-hanging-out shots—I sent her an email and waited for her thunderous approval. Which came within thirty minutes: "Let's meet for lunch tomorrow at Urth Café."

My heart sank as I stared at the computer screen. Everyone in Hollywood is quick to praise you and tell you how ahhmazing you are out of fear that you might actually be important to them one day. Marianne was not like most of the industry suits—she was not afraid to have an opinion and share it. Her lack of praise or criticism in this moment could only mean one thing: Indifference—which is never a good thing for a would-be celebrity.

The following afternoon I parked my 1998 convertible Chevy Cavalier three blocks from the restaurant in order to avoid the $5 fee and luxury car line at the valet. Once inside the terribly trendy but delicious Los Angeles hotspot, I gave myself one mission: Find a prime seat. Marianne was fussy and demanded to be in the middle of everything fabulous. The food really is tasty, but let's face facts: Models, screenwriters, unemployed actors and Europeans all gathered at Urth Café to be seen—like going to the Playboy Mansion.

Marianne made a fashionably late—but still noticeable—entrance wearing a pink, orange and red floral patterned silk blouse neatly tucked into a white spandex micro-skirt that not even Kate Hudson could pull off. Literally, it was that tight. Her faux hair was backcombed and sprayed with so much aerosol the fumes were still visible. She wore a sensible turquoise mule, which matched the color of the eye shadow she had over-applied. Her red lips downplayed the brilliant white gleam of her porcelain veneers that lit a pathway directly to the table I scored in the center of it all. She maneuvered her way through the young and gorgeous, stopping occasionally to interject her unsolicited comments to those foolish enough to make direct eye contact with her—the whole time her Tiffany's charm bracelet rattled against her life-alert band creating the uncomfortable sound of Father Time.

I stood and made my way toward her, to receive her with a big hug and double air kisses. She dropped down into the chair and began gossiping. She was not quiet, or nice, about the observations she made, most of which were painfully accurate. It was remarkable how gifted she was at recognizing the strengths and weakness of others, while remaining utterly unaware of her own.

After discussing the latest movies, sharing a laugh over the most recent celebrity scandals and disputing Catherine Zeta-Jones' real age (Marianne was sure that IMDb had it listed wrong), we began to talk shop.

Marianne pulled out a stack of 5x7 photos. She printed out every last one of my headshots and began to spread them out on the table. For a second I thought we were going to decoupage the table or at least play a short match game. Instead, Marianne started sharing her feedback.

She had several categories for her selection process, and while I can't remember them all, I do remember that they were particular, precise, and politically incorrect. She stacked several piles, pulled out her proof-magnifier, leaned forward and went to work.

"Overall I think these are splendid shots. You look very comfortable in front of the camera."

"Thank you Marianne. That's nice to hear."

"You obviously realize that you're no Brad Pitt, but you have strong features, a bright smile, and charisma—which is hard to fake."

"Oh good, well I'm just happy to know that you don't completely hate the photos."

"Why on Earth would you think that?"

"Well, it's just, you know—you didn't really say much when you got my email with the link, so I was preparing for the worst."

"I never give feedback until I've seen all of the digital photos blown up; this way I can really compare images and find the perfect shot."

"Of course, that makes sense."

I watched as Marianne rearranged the photos, occasionally picking one up and then holding it at arm's distance from her face, pulling it in and out slowly, as if she was manipulating the focus on a camera lens. She carefully studied every photo, and would place two seemingly identical shots in front of me and explain why the shots were so drastically different.

"I love the expression in this shot, but I think your posture is more inviting in the other—we might be able to have Russell Photoshop these and make it the perfect commercial shot!"

In my head I'm thinking, they're literally the exact same shot; I wouldn't be surprised if she mistakenly hit the print button twice. Nevertheless, I acknowledged her "insight" and went along with the charade. I'm confident that the would-be actor/models who were sat at the table next to us thought they were being *Punk'd*.

After two hours, three fresh-squeezed lemonades, a wheatgrass smoothie and a shared curry chicken salad, she had narrowed her selection down to six photos: two commercial shots, two theatrical (more dramatic) and two "personality" shots—which according to her, could "go either way."

The process was arduous and I was relieved when she gave me the green light to have the final six blown up into 8x10 proofs for a second pass. She collected the remaining pile of unwanted mugshots and handed them to me—she assured me that they make sensational gifts for loved ones and the perfect postcards to promote myself to industry professionals. (This was a softer side I would never have expected.)

As she picked pebble-sized chunks of chicken from her teeth (which I had been ignoring for over an hour) she rambled on about making sure she left with plenty of time to make it to Barry's Bootcamp. I assumed she told people she was heading to boot camp, but she was more likely going to Richard Simmons' gym in Beverly Hills. Marianne stuck me more as a *Sweatin' to the Oldies* gal vs. a *Drop It Like It's Hot* chick, but I didn't take the bait.

"Oh, one more thing," she said nonchalantly. "Remind me to give you the name of a marvelous plastic surgeon. He's in Beverly Hills, and all of the stars go to him."

"Ha! You're so Hollywood," I snorted, positive that she was jokingly referencing a conversation that we had earlier in the meeting.

"No, I'm just honest. *We* need to have that mole "looked" at. My *guy* (everyone in Los Angeles has a "guy") is the best in town, and we need to get that mole removed."

Suddenly I felt my heart in my balls. I hadn't thought about my mole in years. Sure, I would get the occasional stare from a three-year-old or an adult who was raised without manners, but aren't we past this?

"I have my mole checked regularly for cancer, and so far I'm good!" I tried to brush it off and move on.

"No darling, you are not good. That mole is going to cause us to lose jobs. You have to trust me on this. I'll call you with his number this evening."

With that, she gave me a double air kiss and sashayed away through the Euro-sexy crowd.

I got home and started obsessing. I could recall a handful of occasions in the past where someone had made a mountain out of my molehill. Still very green, an acting coach in New York informed me that I would need to get it removed and I reminded her that she was there to help me be a better actor, not advise me on my skin care. Also in New York, I was released from a toothpaste commercial because of Molie, but I didn't give it much consideration. In the same month I had booked two separate commercials and neither brand seemed to care about my growth.

I went to the bathroom and stared in the mirror for hours. I realized that I had become blind to my mole years ago. I accepted it and embraced it as a part of my persona. My mole helped me build character throughout my childhood, and was most certainly the reason I had the sassy flair that people had come to know and expect from me.

Once I could no longer gaze into the mirror at myself in contemplation, I decided that I should call Marianne and tell her that the mole was a deal-breaker. I told myself that my talent and determination should be enough to "make it" in Hollywood—and eventually I would book a huge job and show her she was wrong.

Apparently my mole was a more pressing matter than Barry's Bootcamp, because Marianne beat me to the punch. My phone rang several hours after our meeting, and she didn't waste time.

"Grab a pen and take down this number…"

"About that Marianne, I don't think I want to have my mole removed. I don't want to be one of those Hollywood types who think they have to change everything about themselves in order to work as an actor. Besides my mole is what makes me unique and stand out from the crowd."

"Don't be ridiculous—your personality is what makes you shine, that mole is HIDEOUS!" *Literally.*

"Wow, that's a bit harsh. I'm not sure it's that big a deal." I was feeling desperate and under major attack.

"Honey, that mole *is* a big deal. You want to be a movie star right? (She didn't wait for my reply.) Well, close your eyes and imagine your face on massive movie screens across the country—your mole would take up half of those screens!"

I had momentarily lost my ability to compose a sentence; instead I listened in silent shock.

I've always been adequate at hiding my extremely sensitive nature through comedy, but this was one phone call I didn't know how to get out of. Marianne was not backing down—because I was still young (my early twenties) and fresh on the LA scene again, I wanted to do the right thing.

When I was a child the idea of someone cutting away the pain and suffering from the constant hailstorm of hate from the other kids was enough for me to fake a removal. Now, I was terrified at the thought of allowing a doctor (Beverly Hills, or not) to hack into my face.

The following morning I found myself in the waiting room of Dr. Fancy Pants sitting across from a woman who looked to be in her mid sixties, but was probably in her forties and just had *that* much work done. She avoided eye contact with me for as long as possible, but I was fixated on the black and blue bruises that covered her face. She smiled as I walked past her to turn in my new patient paperwork (which by the way is like signing away your life) and she assured me, "It doesn't hurt as bad as it looks!" I've never witnessed someone so happy about looking annihilated—clearly her meds were working.

Shortly after arriving I was called back into a small but lavish examination room—within five minutes Dr. Fancy Pants was fondling my mole. Poking it, rubbing it, squeezing it, massaging it, and measuring it. If this is what he does for a mole, imagine what a breast exam might look like.

After careful analysis Dr. Fancy Pants was convinced that it was deeply rooted, which was the perfect metaphor for my mole. He continued that he would be able to remove it, but not without a very minor scar, that if treated, would heal without much complication. He confirmed that the mole did not look suspicious but he would send it off to the lab to be screened for skin cancer either way.

Then I asked him the question I ask everyone when I'm confronted with a new thought, and have an expert in front of my face: "What would you do?"

"I can't answer that question. You'll have to decide that on your own. But I will tell you that it is very likely that you may have to have it removed at some point in your life, so it might as well be now, while you're young and your skin is elastic enough to heal."

"If I decide to do this, how long will the procedure take, and once it's over how long until it looks normal?"

Dr. Fancy Pants explained that he would do the surgery in his office operating room with only a local anesthesia, and that the whole event should be less than thirty-five minutes.

He scribbled a few lines across a piece of paper to explain how he would make the incisions and keep the scarring down to a minimum. As he continued to talk, I started to feel the not-so-subtle call to "fix" the other things on my body that had held me back since I was a kid, like my lack of abdominal muscles. In his office for less than an hour, and I was intoxicated with the scent of perfection. This guy was REALLY good at his job. Not just in the operating room, but in the sales room, too.

I scheduled my appointment for the following week and left his office with a pre-surgery care guide and even more documents that required my name in blood.

On the car ride home from Beverly Hills, I called my mom to discuss the idea of removing my mole.

"Hi mom. I've got some big news…"

"Did you book a job?"

"No, not yet—but hopefully soon! That's why I'm calling."

"Oh, what's up?"

"You remember when I was younger and used to beg you to remove my mole? Well, I think I'm finally going to get it taken off."

"What?! No, why would you want to do that?"

I filled in the back story, and then:

"Oh great, you're going to turn into one of those Hollywood phonies! I can't believe you'd even consider changing how God made you."

"Don't bring God into this." Even though my mom grew up in the Catholic Church and raised us the same, she was never a religious person, and would only use this type of defense when she had no valid argument.

"Listen mom, I don't love the idea of removing it either, but if it means more opportunities to work as an actor, I have to go for it."

My dad's reaction on the other hand was exactly the opposite of what I thought it was going to be.

"You've worked so hard to get to this point in your life, if you think it's going to make or break your career, I say go for it. You've always wanted to remove it anyway."

After a week of contemplating my mole massacre, I decided that Marianne was right; my mole does not define me—I called Dr. Fancy Pants to confirm my surgery.

Two days later I arrived at the lush Beverly Hills office. My sixth grade scandal was actually happening and my stomach was in knots. It was too late to change my mind now. After a serious photo shoot capturing every angle of my face, I took one final glance in the mirror before following a nurse into the operating room.

Dr. Fancy Pants was scrubbed in and ready to coach me through my procedure. He began with a cream followed by two injections that rendered my entire face completely numb—which is how I imagine the Cat Lady or Ryan Seacrest must feel every day.

The doctor began cutting into my face about twenty minutes later, and aside from the dreadful sound of someone hacking through gristle and the smell of burning flesh, it was a fairly painless operation.

Once he completed my face augmentation, he covered the wound and instructed me to keep the bandage on for the first four days, after which I should return to his office in order to remove the stitches. He wrote me a prescription for Vicodin and sent me on my way.

The weekend was tough. Like my former closeted self in the high school locker room, I wanted to sneak a peak—of my new mole-less face. The Vicodin was a warm-fuzzy distraction. I sat eagerly as Dr. Fancy Pants removed the piles of gauze from my face. At last, the final bandage was removed, and with a confident smile he turned to the nurse and she smiled back while declaring, "You couldn't have done a better job!"

They had their shtick worked out, because when he handed me the mirror to take my first glance, I froze in horror. What was once a small (okay—pink eraser sized) mole, was now a HUGE scar that ran from the bottom corner of my left nostril to the bottom corner of my lip. It was like a railroad track for snot.

Believe me, there was a lot of snot and tears building up while I sat in his office as he explained how (over time) the scar would heal and be *almost* invisible. With that, he handed me a steroid cream and told me to use it five to six times a day in order to help with the swelling.

As soon as I exited the Beverly Hills butcher, I began sobbing uncontrollably. What had I done? Would I ever look attractive again? Why did I listen to a manager who wears synthetic hair?

Over the following weeks, I followed the doctor's instructions implicitly and to my delight and shock the scar began to fade away. Within two months the Frankenstein-like tracks faded into light pink lines and I started auditioning and booking jobs.

Time passed and like my mole, my relationship with Marianne had vanished. She was right that my birthmark was holding me back, but what I didn't acknowledge until I had it removed, is that the greater gift that Marianne inspired was confidence in myself.

My mole was not an extension of who I am, although it helped me discover my inner character when I was younger. Marianne recognized this. By the time I reached adulthood, I had accepted my mole as a part of me. It defined me in the sense that I had endured adolescence, and I wore it as a badge of honor. In removing the mole, I released the idea that my mole made me unique and became aware that my individualism was not based on what I looked like.

Occasionally I'll catch a glimpse of myself in a mirror and see my mole. Secretly, I miss it. Molie helped me find my voice and enabled me to see past other people's imperfections. My personality does make me unique, but that mole helped me rock my confidence, which is why I keep Molie in a tiny jar beneath my bed, and from time to time I pull him out and stick him on my face as a reminder of how far I've come.

The Art of Catering

Despite having a handful of friends who earned easy money, made fabulous connections, and met their future spouses rubbing elbows with the rich and nasty, I miraculously managed to survive my twenties in New York City without becoming the clichéd actor-turned-cater-waiter. Not that I'm afraid of hard work; I got my hands dirty performing random acts of desperation as a promo model, camp counselor, Pottery Barn sales associate, nanny, and bar mitzvah dancer. I still have day-terrors from the trauma that four hundred privileged thirteen-year-olds can inflict upon a struggling artist. No one could persuade me to get my only pair of Prada shoes scuffed up passing pu-pu platters to people at parties where I *should* have been on the guest list.

When I moved back to Los Angeles, what I lacked in money I overcompensated in determined ambition; I knew I was going to make it big. I continued to live off the unemployment I collected from a show that had closed when I left New York and I was actively auditioning for jobs. I had also started working for a large national talent competition: think *American Idol* meets *So You Think You Can Dance* without the TV cameras (or the talent). I was hardly making ends meet, but in true LA style I kept spending like a movie star.

In La La Land image is everything. How you're perceived plays a big hand in what you will receive. In order to keep up with the demanding lifestyle, I started doing something I had never done before—I used my plastic. Hey, it's LA, everyone believes in plastic. [BEAT] Surgery.

The charge-o-thon started off slow at first. I was only using credit cards for essential items that I didn't have the extra income for: head

157

shots, acting classes, gym membership, gas, food, rent, Gucci pants, a $2000 Yorkshire Terrier, date nights, Disneyland, clubbing, okay it was starting to add up, and before I could control it I was twenty-six thousand dollars in debt.

Penniless and turning thirty—I had to come to terms with my situation. Thanks to a declining economy, there were few opportunities for undiscovered actors. Throw in an organized strike by the Writers' union and the outlook went from "it could happen" to "unless you're Brad Pitt, it's not happening right now." I needed to get a job. It was time to roll up my sleeves and start sweating.

I needed something that would get me back on track financially, without taking me away from my dream of becoming a working actor. As a kid I mowed lawns, but that market has been marvelously maintained by a monopoly that not even Trump could wall out. I was also a babysitter, but (aside from Britney Spears) who wants to pay a thirty-year-old performer twenty dollars an hour, when they can get the neighbor girl to do it for ten? When I turned fifteen, I worked in my grandparents' print shop, gathering papers, collating books, and filing account invoices—but who goes to a print shop anymore?

What am I going to do? I will NOT be a server. I just can't do it again. I was nineteen when a disgruntled customer spat a mouthful of food on me, to validate the fact that his food was "colder than Ann Coulter's soul", which was the end of my six month stint as a part-time server in a breakfast restaurant in Chicago.

After serious contemplation I was left with two options: I could get into the porn industry or I could take up my friend's offer to work private events as a cater-waiter. I'd like to point out that either job would mean I would be earning an income while getting screwed, but at least with porn it might feel good, too. I didn't want my first extreme close up to include a graphic money shot, so with a heavy heart I accepted the latter position.

I phoned my friend Helen and told her I would take the job. Her misplaced enthusiasm was enough to give me a second thought: "Why are you so thrilled that I said yes?"

"Because it's always nice to have a friend in Hell." She said without a trace of humor or irony.

I could actually taste the bitter shame of my state of affairs as I approached the impeccably manicured rolling lawns and deeply rooted Magnolia trees that surrounded the mansion grounds in the prestigious Hancock Park area of Los Angeles. Worse than a trip to the doctor when you know something is wrong, but are living in denial, I was trying to suppress the truth: I'm accustomed to performing or attending parties thrown in houses like this; now I'm the help.

I rang the doorbell. After waiting for several minutes the door opened to reveal a half-dressed brash woman with curlers in her hair and nothing but concealer under her eyes. Imagine a mop-headed, felt-faced, curvy creature from *Fraggle Rock* trying to look like Sarah Jessica Parker. She greeted me with arms wide open, and a loud Hel-LLO in a thick Australian dialect. Upon embracing me in a hug (where she unapologetically felt me up) she invited me in.

I walked through the ornate wrought iron French doors into a living room that was the size of an NBA court. The dark hardwood floors were very easy to take in, because there wasn't any furniture. Lauren Cosgrove (the raccoon-like-Muppet) led me down the side hallway, which passed a galley bar and fed into the kitchen where Helen stood desperately awaiting my arrival.

"Oh, good, you're here. Thanks Lauren, I'll catch him up with what we're doing."

"Wonderful, and don't forget to show him where we need those buckets of ice moved before the party starts. . ." Lauren let the last four words trail off to remain authoritative but aloof.

"What do you need?" I said to Helen while Lauren was still in earshot. I've always been an overachieving hustler, and I get a lot accomplished in a short amount of time, but I'm not afraid to make sure the people in charge know my value. The going rate at the time was twenty-five dollars an hour, and all the food and wine I could consume between waiting on party guests.

Helen casually walked over to me with an egregious look on her face. "This is going to be a Shit-Show! I don't even know where to begin. In less than an hour, 50 six-year-olds and their parents will be here. *She* wants to serve two specialty cocktails… at a kids' party?! We don't even have enough glasses, which means one of us will have to be in here washing while the other one serves."

Helen took a brief pause from complaining to come up for air. That's when I found my opportunity to get the facts: "Why is the place empty?"

"What?"

"Why is there so little furniture in this house? I thought you said they had a lot of money?"

"We're understaffed and facing people in less than thirty minutes, and that's all you care about?"

"Helen, we'll be fine. I'll smile at everyone, rave about how brilliant their last project was, and act like they're the most important thing on the planet when I deliver their alcohol. Let's be honest, once they're two glasses in they won't care about us anyway."

"Great plan. Do you want a glass of wine?" Helen recovered quickly from her panic and picked up the very full glass of wine that she had hidden behind a toaster oven.

"Yes. And please tell me what her story is!"

"I don't know. She collects art. Or sells it, or something... I don't know. Her husband is a fancy-pants music executive and I'm sure that's where the real money comes from."

I checked out of the conversation once I realized how miserable Helen was, and I decided to explore the surroundings. If I have to spend my day serving rich bald men and their latest anorexic arm candy, with a sprinkle of former sitcom stars from the eighties I'm going to find every emergency exit and hiding place in this house in case I need to make a break for it.

"I'll be right back." With that I was out of the kitchen and making my way into what should have been the dining room.

Where one would expect an overpriced luxury table, I attempted to digest what looked like a heap of scrap metal and computer parts. The only thing separating the pile of "art" from the rest of the room was a piece of nylon white rope, which protected the maid from mistakenly throwing out the garbage. I'm not someone who ordinarily or carelessly passes judgment of another artist's work, but this looked less like a work of art and more like a Silicon Valley tech giant's angry failed prototype pile. At best, it was a poor man's replica of something more interesting I'd seen at the MOCA years earlier.

As I snaked through the mazelike house two things became crystal clear: 1.) There was "art" randomly plopped throughout the house, and 2.) This shindig was more than a birthday party for Lauren's daughter; this was an art gallery birthday bombardment.

I found my way back to the kitchen and inquired, "Helen, how did you come to know Lauren again?"

Before responding, Helen picked up a fresh glass of wine and took a hearty drink. "Craig met Lauren at a dinner party, and I think he bought a piece of art from her?"

Now it all made sense. Craig is a dear friend of Helen's. He's a handsome, gay man and well-known photographer who comes from East Coast old money.

"Hellooooo?! Are you going to help me cut these lemons? We've still got to figure out our specialty cocktails." Helen always gets a little edgy when it comes to planning, especially if it involves waiting on people.

"Margaritas and Martinis?!" I offer a practical, delicious solution to manage her nerves.

"Really? Doesn't it seem a little boring?"

"Helen, it's a children's birthday party and we're serving alcohol. I don't think that falls into the category of boring. In some states it's classified as child endangerment."

Just as I finished my rant, Lauren walked in. "Have we decided on drinks?"

"Actually, we just decided on the menu: margaritas with fresh squeezed lime juice and agave or a classic Martini."

"Darling, that sounds magnificent. Just be sure not to over serve anyone! We want them to enjoy themselves, but let's not forget it's a birthday party for my gorgeous little angel."

Lauren floated out of the kitchen to greet the lifeguard whom she hired to make sure no children (or drunk adults) drowned in her pool.

We finished the last of the prep work just as the doorbell rang. Ladies and gentlemen break out your checkbooks, it's time to buy some art. From that moment on, Helen and I worked non-stop; there were only two of us, and two hundred guests. We could not keep up. Every time we turned the corner an annoying socialite was complaining about an empty glass. We on the other hand continued habitually drinking whatever alcohol we could find between every stop we made to or from the kitchen. At one point a balding, overweight, powerful man demanded that I stop what I was doing in order to get him something from Lauren's private reserve.

Slightly tipsy and with both arms full of trash, empty glasses, and an ashtray full of butts, I responded, "Sir, I have no idea what you are referring to, but I'm happy to get you another cocktail as soon as I take care of this." Indicating the balancing act that I was moments away from losing.

"I don't know why you're implying that Lauren and Paul don't have a better selection of top shelf alcohol. I'm a very *personal* friend and I happen to know that in their wine cellar..."

"Let me stop you right there. I'm not implying anything. This is my first time working for Lauren. I'm sure she has plenty of top shelf alcohol for you. I don't know where she keeps it. Thankfully, you're a *very personal friend* of Lauren's, so I encourage you to let her know that you're unhappy with the selection she's planned for today. I imagine she'll hook you up." I vanished like David Copperfield into the side hallway, which I had scouted earlier for this precise reason.

Despite our best efforts to keep guests out of the kitchen, a parade of D-list famous faces rolled up to the imported Carrera marble island in search of "something stronger to drink." Helen and I knew what they were really looking for was more food because they had been smoking medical grade marijuana and had the munchies. If Lauren was going for an upscale version of Jimmy Buffet's Margaritaville, mission accomplished.

The last of the guests made their way toward the front entrance as I chugged the remaining mixture of tequila, agave, and lime juice. I was ready for this moment in my life to be over.

Lauren walked into the kitchen as if she'd been working in a sweatshop in a third world country. "I. Am. So. Exhausted."

I kept my mouth shut and smiled.

"You guys were brilliant. I know *we* weren't expecting that many guests (a bold lie), but you handled it like pros!"

Again, I kept my mouth shut and glared at Helen.

"You don't have to finish up with those dishes, I'll have Rita do them tomorrow."

"Are you sure? We don't mind." Helen was always trying to do the right thing.

I wanted to strangle Helen.

"No, it's quite alright. How much do I owe you?"

"I think we agreed on two-hundred and fifty dollars." Helen also hates dealing with money.

Lauren reached into her Louis Vuitton fanny pack and pulled out six hundred dollars. She divided the bills up and handed us each half. "I threw in a little tip, because there was more work than we expected."

Helen and I reached for the cash and thanked her. We gushed over how adorable her daughter was. We gossiped about how hot the lifeguard was. And we raved about how delightful the horrible human beings she referred to as "friends" were.

Lauren asked us to mark our calendar for a date the following month as we were leaving. Caught off guard and unable to fully process the demand, we obliged. We had just agreed to work another understaffed—adult only—dinner party.

Days leading up to our sixth dinner party I tried to catch a cold. The only way I could turn down money at this point in my debt was if I was laid up in a bed, on the verge of death with no hope of survival. For this party, Lauren had requested three more cater-waiters to work with us. With a lot of begging, bribing, and empty promises, Helen and I convinced three of our closest friends to endure the torture.

The night of the party, Helen called and informed me that she would be picking us up an hour before our call time in order to buy ice. Already I was raging over the fact that we had to run errands for this lackadaisical, spoon-fed, FAUX-cialite. Doesn't she have a maid that handles her shopping?

Helen stopped the car outside of the heavenly sized gates, which marked the entrance to my personal perdition. I grabbed the ice that was already half melted, and made my way down the graveled pathway. Abandoning all of my manners or etiquette, I walked through the open doors and directly to the bar, dropped the semi-frozen water into the sink, and poured myself a glass of chilled white wine. Lauren greeted me out of nowhere like the host from *How To Catch A Predator*, with a familiar and still very inappropriate groping followed by two air kisses. Once she was done fondling me, she asked me to gather the other "helpers" into the kitchen so she could explain her game plan.

Helen, Jeff, Brooke, Amy and I sat around a buffet table in a corner of her kitchen awaiting her master plan. Mountains of serving platters, glassware, and bags of groceries dominated the landscape. This was going to be *the* Shit-Show to end all Shit-Shows.

Lauren made her entrance while talking. "Do any of you know how to follow a recipe?" Her budget no longer included a private chef.

Like a true leader I began delegating. I offered up my husband: "Jeff is an exceptional cook and follows recipes with the excellence you'd expect on *Top Chef.*"

"Marvelous! We'll be serving beef tenderloin, potatoes au gratin, and grilled asparagus."

Lauren led Jeff to the prep station in her massive, yet cumbersome galley kitchen where a nine-hundred-dollar cut of meat—it may have been half a cow—laid wrapped in butcher paper. She began to explain in great detail exactly how she wanted everything cooked. Following her rapid-fire line of directions she turned to the rest of us and said, "The rest of you can decide who's serving and who will help in the kitchen. Oh, and does anyone know how to roll a joint?"

Once more, I sacrificed a friend, "Brooke is an expert."

"Perfect. Brooke, can you please meet me in the dining room in ten minutes?"

I watched Brooke's eyes roll in my direction as Lauren exited the kitchen. We all gathered around Jeff and tried to devise a plan. No one signed up to be a chef. Let the games begin!

Jeff, the resourceful pro that he is, quickly organized the food in order of cook time. He delegated tasks to his sous-chef, Helen and asked if Amy could assist him with clean up. Because Brooke and I were the most social of our group (and really unhappy in a kitchen) we decided to take the reigns of cocktails and passing food. Our work was cut out for us and we were ready. Alas, the oven was not.

Indulge me while I backtrack. I neglected to mention that since our last catering gig, Lauren and her family had "scaled back" their lifestyle. Even the new-money gallery owner and her pop-producing husband had to face the music, and 2008 did not offer a stellar playlist for anyone.

They sold their nearly empty mansion and moved into a passé Hancock Park Adjacent rental house. Despite the downfall of the U. S. economy, the Cosgroves continued to throw lavish parties. They managed to maintain the illusion of wealth and success within their network of clients, who were primarily established society or old money. But nobody was buying art, and behind the scenes the rented walls were crumbling. The oven was just one of the many neglected luxuries.

Guests were scheduled to arrive in less than twenty minutes; we stared at the oven waiting for signs of life. Jeff began to panic. "How in hell am I supposed to make a dinner from scratch for sixty people without an oven?"

As much as I wanted to help him out, Brooke and I were busy prepping limes, hand washing the stemware, carrying boxes of wine from the cellar, arranging flowers throughout the house, and Brooke was already fifteen minutes late to marijuana rolling. I grabbed a bottle of whiskey, poured a round of shots and wished my crew good luck.

The doorbell rang moments later. With a smile and a bottle of Veuve Clicquot, I greeted the cheerless couple and encouraged them to enjoy their champagne by the fireplace. There was an awkward tension—the first to arrive are always the worst. Through their forced smiles, I could tell that they had been fighting, but I was not their marriage counselor and I had lime wedges to cut, so I was off. As I turned to walk away I heard the mousey woman ask, "Is Lauren around?"

"She should be down momentarily," I lied. Lauren was still in her robe supervising the wacky weed rollup.

"Will there be music at this *party?*" The irritated man grunted.

"Yes, of course, once the party *starts*, there will be a lively playlist." I couldn't help shaming them for their early arrival, which was always a sure sign of desperation in LA.

I joined Brooke in Lauren's sitting room to lend my hand with the joint assembly line. Lauren was putting the finishing touches on her make-up and confessed that there might be more people than she anticipated. Big surprise, her eye make-up and headcounts were always overindulgent.

"We'll make it work," she declared before walking out of the room to greet her eager arrivals.

Back in the Hell's kitchen, Jeff, Helen, and Amy masterfully rigged the oven to cook the most expensive meat I've seen in my life (and I lived in New York City), charred four pounds of asparagus, and peeled sixty potatoes with enough time to polish off two bottles of wine.

Brooke and I joined the rest of the group with enough time to argue over how to slice a lime. The mood gets sour when you task two know-it-alls with any procedure involving a knife. Lauren barged into the kitchen to add more bitter juice: "I'm afraid we're going to have to make room for twenty more."

"I'm afraid, too!" I blurted out before thinking. Wine and (many) shots of Patron have played a featured role in my mood swing. Usually the guest count is off by one or two couples max and we'd cram them in on the end of the table and call it a day. That technique was not going to work this time. The already overcrowded table spanned the length of her entire empty dining and living rooms, leaving little space to hold your breath and turn to the side as you walked around. It was like present-day Oprah trying to squeeze back into the skinny jeans she wore on her first weight loss reveal circa 1988. Guests had been pinched into a section of the table where no one could even pick up their forks to eat without violating serious boundaries.

Lauren unceasingly tried to set a lavish table and it always ended up looking like something Martha Stewart would fire a mid-level design executive for. Evident to every guest with eyes that they were an afterthought, they'd continue to show up, drink her fancy wine and top shelf alcohol, and shell out for artwork that was less Renoir and more Ronald McArtist.

The early arrivals were now adequately lubricated and all of the usual characters descended upon us like mini-tragedies that unfold through a Greek chorus. We liked to refer to *these* people as the guest stars in Lauren's sitcom. Horrifically, we were the extras in this dramedy that you'd assuredly binge on Netflix; and our show lasted much longer than thirty minutes. The worst part was when one of her famous friends would sashay into the kitchen and start making requests. They always approached us as if they knew us and we were BFF's. You had to respond swiftly, fearlessly, and directly with these guests; my top three witty comebacks were:

1. I know you from TV, but we are not friends—unless you'd like to introduce me to your agent after this party?

2. I don't care if you're on an all vegan diet to prepare for a part in a television movie for Hallmark. We don't have a vegan option. Talk to your hostess (not her help) for a solution.

3. If I'm being totally honest, you're not a very kind person and your performances to date have been remarkably unwatchable, which is not really helping your situation.

Then, I would start talking about how phenomenal one of their co-stars is and how rewarding it must be to work with them; this would usually do the trick. Occasionally (after loads of alcohol) they would begin spilling the juicy details of a fellow thespian. The goal was to get them out of the serving area, so that we could continue drinking Lauren's top shelf alcohol.

Once all seventy-five guests were seated at a table for ten, the service began. As we moved through the main course, into cheese plates and then desserts, the crowed began to calm down. The handcrafted joints that were passed around the table helped ease the tension and allowed us time in the kitchen to clean dishes, drink more, and gossip about what we overheard around the table. Paul and Lauren's lack of love life was always our appetizer, who cheated on whom our main course, and which celebrity's offspring was failing kindergarten our devious dessert.

Despite the seriously failing economy, Lauren continued to host lavish parties every two or three months, each one with less production value than the last. The cutbacks started off small. Instead of lighting fifty white tapper candles throughout the house, she'd set out ten or fifteen at a time, and instruct us to extinguish them after the first hour. Rather than buying cases of wine and champagne, she'd ask us to stretch ten bottles during the course of an evening, which would usually be plenty for a dinner party, but her guests had become accustomed to a "no empty glass" policy. Toward the end she was buying pre-made bulk food from Costco and her deluxe guests were none the wiser.

Lauren was cutting corners everywhere she could, so it came as no surprise to us that she was going to "scale back" on our catering team. She would hire three people and have one person show up an hour earlier to do all of the prep work on their own. She would cut two people while guests were still at the party and have one person do the clean up. At the end of an evening we would gather in her kitchen and rather than cash, she would hand us a check. Her buy-in-bulk budget was reflected in the dollar amount of our checks and there was no sign of a tip.

On the second to last party that we worked for her, she decided to pull out all of the stops. She came into a windfall of money and she couldn't wait to blow it. The whole catering team was reunited, the food was stellar, the alcohol flowed freely, and the party raged on until one in the morning. When the last of the guests slurred their drunken goodnights, we piled into the kitchen ready to collect a fat paycheck.

To our dismay, Lauren—in her dazed and drunken stupor—declared that she was unable to locate her checkbook. Interestingly, she had no trouble locating my ass just moments before. This had never happened before and we were all caught off guard.

Begrudgingly, we wrote our addresses down on a piece of butcher paper and handed it to Lauren's assistant as instructed. Lauren gave each of us that oh-so-fabulous double air kiss and a hug, and promised to send our check out first thing in the morning. She'd always paid us, so we had no reason to believe this would be an issue. Our checks arrived two days later, sans tip.

I was living paycheck-to-paycheck and desperate for money, so I took my check to the fancy bank from which it was drawn on, to cash it. I handed the "private banker" my check and driver's license and waited for her to hand over my cash. Shocker, there was an "issue". The teller called over her manager to explain to me that they could not cash the check.

"I don't understand? I called ahead to confirm that I didn't need an account here in order to cash my check?"

"That's correct sir, you don't need an account. However, we're unable to cash this check at the moment." The manager's face said everything I needed to know, but I had to ask anyways.

"Are you telling me that there isn't enough money in her account to cover a three-hundred dollar check?"

"We're not at liberty to discuss our clients' personal affairs, but I can tell you that if you wait three weeks, we should be able to cash this for you."

Unbelievable. Money-bags-party-hostess extraordinaire threw a party she couldn't afford. I thought only artists did that, not the gallery owners too.

Three weeks later I returned to the bank and cashed the check. I vowed I would never work at a Lauren Cosgrove party again.

It's a well-known fact that whenever you vow never to do something again, the universe forces you to eat your words. In my case, it came in the form of a phone call from my accountant. I miscalculated how much I was going to owe on my taxes, and I needed to come up with an extra five hundred dollars or Uncle Sam was going to stick more than a feather in my cap.

Like a heroin junky looking for his next fix, I called Helen and agreed to another dinner party disaster; never stopping to consider that the needle was probably dirty.

The night was no different than any of Lauren's previous parties; we were understaffed, overworked, and bitter. One perk was that most of her guests had become so accustomed to our presence that they included us in conversation as we made our rounds.

Halfway through the evening the catering crew gathered in a hidden corner of the house to toast with a bottle of Jose Cuervo Anejo Reserva De La Familia that we found while searching for crystal stemware at the command of Lauren. We knew it wasn't right to drink a two hundred dollar bottle of tequila without at least inviting our hostess to drink her alcohol with us, but we figured she'd want us to enjoy it in lieu of a tip for the last three parties. After our second glass of the smooth, complex, one-of-a-kind tequila I looked around at all of the new artwork that was displayed so beautifully (for a change). I looked at my friends and made a declaration: "If she doesn't pay us in cash tonight, be prepared to grab a painting and start walking; don't stop until we get to the car. We're leaving with our money, even if it's in the form of up-and-coming art."

My friends started laughing. I was half joking. I started exploring how the art was mounted on the walls.

The guests had long since left and we had been busy cleaning dishes, restocking wine glasses, and drinking more tequila. It was late and we were ready to split but Lauren was nowhere to be found.

We searched high and low, until I approached the one room I never expected her to be in—her daughter's. There she was, hiding in plain sight. Reading a book to her daughter—probably a first for both of them—and just as I was about to ask her for our check, she cut me off. "I'm having a moment with my daughter. I will send your checks in the mail tomorrow."

The first week came and went and we didn't receive our checks. Not cool, but nothing to get alarmed over, Lauren has always paid us. She would never stiff us; we have several very *important* mutual friends in common. Toward the end of the second week I started to get frustrated. What a cliché, Lauren was a typical nouveau riche gallery owner keeping "the help" waiting for their money. As eager as she was to sell a piece of artwork to pad her pocket book and help one of her miserably broke artists, she refused to accept that the *actors* serving her guest were just as anguished and equally impoverished. When we reached the end of the third week without a payment, I was flat out pissed.

Until this point, Helen had been our catering agent. She was the person who would reach out to Lauren or her assistant Tom if there were a question or concern. I called Helen. "Helen, what is going on? It's been over three weeks and I *need* my money."

"I spoke with Tom, Lauren's assistant who was recently promoted to un-paid 'partner,' and he said that the checks have been sent out."

I couldn't help but snort, "Really, the check's in the mail? That's the line they're leading with? Did he say why there's been a three week delay?"

"I didn't ask, but I know that Lauren has been out of town, so that might be why."

I could hear the trepidation in Helen's response. She truly despises this type of engagement, so I decided I was going to have to take matters into my own hands.

"Okay, well let's keep our fingers crossed. If they've sent the checks, we should receive them today or tomorrow!"

As soon as I hung up the phone, I knew it was time to take matters into my own hands. I used to have a temper as devastating as one of the *Real Housewives of Beverly Hills* traveling without their make-up artist. Extensive amounts of yoga and endless self-help books inspired me to stay calm and reach out in a civilized manner.

Lauren's *partner* offered the same canned response I had heard from Helen moments before; still I couldn't help but push the matter further. "I understand that Lauren has been out of town, but why wasn't the check sent the day following our event, as promised?"

Tom answered casually, "It was just an oversight. We're really sorry, but I assure you that will receive your check by tomorrow at the latest."

Not satisfied, I decided to twist the knife deeper, "Will we be able to cash it when we receive it, or will we have to wait another three weeks for the check to clear, like last time?"

"No, there will be no issues." Tom was quick to hang up the phone.

Four days later my mailbox was still empty. My agitation had evolved into aggression and I was convinced that Lauren was going to try to get out of paying us for our work.

On day six—after nearly thirty voice messages—Tom picked up the phone. His exasperated voice indicated that my relentless outreach was taking its toll. He offered a pathetic excuse about confusion at the office and assured me that money was on the way.

"Tom, I know there was no miscommunication, because I know that Lauren's *office* is her bedroom. Save the cover up. I just want to know that my check will be in my mailbox within two days. Are you telling me that there will not be a further delay?"

"I promise."

Tom was a fellow gay and I really wanted to believe him. I waited for the check in the same way that I anticipate another relevant album from Madonna; we all want it to come but the odds are not in our favor. Another week passed.

Despite the pleas from the catering crew, I summoned my inner rage—that I spent most of my childhood suppressing—jumped into my used Chevy Cavalier and drove to Lauren's house. My blood was near boiling as I drove my not-cool-teal-green convertible through West Hollywood down Crescent Heights over to Beverly and into Hancock Park. My face was wrenched as I snorted nasty phrases that I was practicing in my rearview mirror at every stoplight. I've been burned by people before—but I've never gone down without a fight, and I certainly wasn't going to let this bourgeois friend of a friend get away with screwing me out of the money I worked for because she thinks I'm just a nobody in this town.

One red light after another—I took it as a sign from the universe that I needed to calm down. Deep breaths and a clear head would go further than a childish outburst.

I wish I had my iPhone ready to capture the look on Tom's face as he answered Lauren's door. Aliens having sex with the ghost of Picasso would have been less of a jolt.

"Matthew, what are you doing here?"

"Hey Tom, I think it's pretty obvious why I'm here—I'd like to collect our checks."

"I wish you would have called, I could have saved you the trip. We just sent the checks out this morning."

"Please don't take this personally, Tom, but I don't believe you. Also, I don't care. I'm not leaving here until I have a check in my hand. It's December 22nd and seven weeks since we worked the party. I leave town tomorrow for the holiday. I seriously doubt that Lauren would attempt this stunt with any of her other vendors."

Tom's face was a shade of red that I thought only existed on cartoons. "Matthew, I don't know what to say? I'm so embarrassed—I'll see if Lauren will re-write the check."

"Thanks Tom, there's not much to say at this point. I don't appreciate being lied to. I just want my money."

Tom nodded, "I'll be right back." He left the door cracked open enough for me to hear a muffled dialogue. I could tell that Lauren was heated, but I couldn't distinguish the bitter words she was spewing.

He returned with his head hung low and a check in his hand. Mission accomplished. When he handed me the check, I glanced to notice that once again there was no tip. I wished him a happy holiday, jumped into my car, and drove straight to Lauren's bank.

I raced through Beverly Hills to make sure I got to the bank before they closed. If I didn't cash this check before my Christmas vacation in Colorado, I would have no money to buy presents for my family. I would be Screwged!

With only twenty minutes left in their work day, the bank tellers were already counting their drawers and cashed out mentally. I walked up to the red velvet rope (everything in Beverly Hills is a VIP event) and waited patiently for the two remaining bankers to discontinue their reenactment of the company holiday party. Annoyed they had to work, they acknowledged my presence and waved me to the window. I grabbed the pen, endorsed the back of the check and handed it over, "I'd like to cash this please."

The teller took the check and started typing on her computer. I observed her face as she continued to type, and noticed that she kept glancing at the check and then back at me. She paused, walked away from the computer with my check and huddled in a corner with a smartly dressed woman who looked slightly out of place. After several minutes, both women walked toward me, pantsuit in the lead, "Sir, I'm afraid we have a problem. The date is incorrect on this check."

"No it isn't, I checked it before I left—she just handed me that check ten minutes ago."

"I'm terribly sorry sir, the month and date are correct, but it's dated for a year from today."

"You. Have. Got. To. Be. FUCKING. KIDDING. ME!!! I can't believe she would do that." With every word more poison escaped.

"Mr. Shaffer, unfortunately there is nothing we can do."

"Oh, yes there is. I'd like you to call her and tell her that if she doesn't explain that she's made an incredible mistake and authorize this payment, she's going to see me back at her rented house with a police escort in ten minutes. Do you understand?"

The intelligent and well-dressed executive processed my tone and urgency. I could tell that she was on my side, and though it was against the bank's policy, she agreed to call her. She stepped away from the window and walked back to the corner, where she proceeded to make the phone call.

After what felt like an hour of nodding, she returned to the window. "Mrs. Cosgrove explained that she had indeed made a mistake and we will be happy to cash the check for you."

"That is wonderful news! Thank you for saving Christmas."

Money in my pocket and my head held high, I walked to my piece-of-shit car and drove back to my apartment. On the ride home, I conference called the rest of my catering team to share the story. I explained that I tried to collect their checks to no avail, but not to expect them anytime soon. When they finally come—I continued—plan on waiting a year to cash them.

That was the last time I worked for Lauren Cosgrove. Our paths would cross from time to time in certain social circles; she would do her best to avoid making contact with me and I would go out of my way to make sure we were forced to engage.

A few years ago I was invited to a lavish dinner party thrown by a host who hired the appropriate amount of catering staff. In between courses, I heard that Lauren was going through a nasty divorce and had to move into a two-bedroom apartment on the outskirts of Hancock Park.

I sympathized for her beautiful children, but I did not shed a tear for Lauren. She painted herself into an impossible position. Like the art that once hung from her rented walls, she was a lackluster imitation of something brilliant. She saw herself as a Degas, but she was nothing more than a poster you'd find in a Z Gallerie. Where true artists cling to integrity, she relied on cheap tricks and post-dated checks. When others were honest, she played dress-up in well-worn couture. In many ways, I could relate to her need to fit in, but I could never understand her inability to comprehend what all of her guests had always known: her home, artwork, and personality lacked authenticity. Working for Lauren reminded me that no amount of money could ever replace the wealth of knowing and accepting yourself.

Only in LA: The 405

After spending an adventurous day at the Happiest Place on Earth, Jeff and I had reached our brim of lines, crying kids, checking out hot dads, and consuming overpriced, flavor enhanced junk food.

I love a parade. Jeff is less of a fan. We compromised and followed behind the *Paint the Night* parade as it slithered down Main Street USA. When the last float carrying the star of the show, Mickey Mouse, finished the loop near the exit of the park, Jeff and I busted into a jazzy dance routine through the turnstile, which put those young Disney dancers to shame.

We continued to chaîné turn across crowded Downtown Disney until we arrived at the Mickey & Friends parking structure—which is roughly the size of England. We ascended to the highest level of the towering island of stacked cars just in time to watch the magical fireworks display illuminate the balmy Orange County sky.

When the dazzling light show ended we continued the trek to our section, Mickey E8 and found my 1998 teal green Chevy Cavalier convertible. It was the ideal night to drive with the top down. Who cares if it gets a little windy or loud on the freeway? You shouldn't drive a convertible in Southern California if you're not going to use it. We jumped in the car, dropped the ragtop, buckled up and hit the road.

Wind in our hair and the radio cranked to KOST 103.5—California's go-to soft rock hits station—we flew up the 5 freeway until we hit traffic approaching the 10 interchange. Hoping to avoid further delays I made a split-second decision to forgo our original route.

Similar to one of the rollercoasters we had just been on at Disneyland, I zipped in and out of traffic, cut over to the right lane and merged onto the 10 west. Rounding the corner of the onramp sent an epic rush of adrenaline; Jeff was clutching the rim of the window as if he might actually be catapulted from the car.

Merging onto the freeway in Los Angeles can be a life-threatening ordeal. You must approach the entrance with the right amount of confidence and speed, while remaining alert and prepared to slam on your brakes at any moment based on the type of drivers you will encounter.

You have the drivers who are terrified of the freeway, so they stay in the slow lane and cause major difficulty for anyone traveling faster than 35 MPH as they approach. There are those who don't want to go faster than the speed limit, but don't want you to pass them either. They piss me off because in addition to cock blocking you from advancing on the road, they tend to be responsible for most of the accidents. There are drunk drivers. Drivers who eat, talk on their cell phones, read scripts, shave, or apply make-up while driving. There are angry drivers; their rage is exposed through their horn or as they cut you off while flipping you the bird. Then you have tourists, who clearly don't know how to operate the rental car navigation system. You also have to watch out for the speed demons. These are the drivers who have a death wish or a failed dream of driving for NASCAR; and don't give a shit about other peoples' safety or about getting a ticket. Motorcycle drivers and semi-truck drivers who add the element of surprise, danger, and a sexy scruffy beard. Finally, there are those assholes that are just looking to cause trouble.

My always enforcing father drilled the importance of scanning the road and checking my rearview mirror regularly, and it was during one of my routine safety glances that I saw one of the aforementioned jerkwads creeping up on the passenger side of my car. Jeff and I had thought that our journey reached its peak earlier in the evening on Space Mountain, but we were about to discover that our adventure was just beginning.

We were trickling along the Santa Monica freeway into a sea of red brake lights that stretched out in front of us beyond the horizon. Behind me, there was nothing but a wake of white headlights.

A black Lincoln Town car abruptly jerked back and forth through cars like a shark until it was side-by-side to my Chevy. The right shoulder bottlenecked, forcing the predator to slam on his brakes to avoid hitting me or speed up and try to cut me off.

I hate bullies—especially vehicular intimidators—so out of principal I wouldn't let him over. "Hey buddy! You can wait your turn like everybody else!" I yelled aloud knowing that the sound wouldn't carry through his tinted black windows. Jeff begged me not to lose my temper, but it was too late.

The livery car driver decided to ram his driver's side front end into the passenger's backend of my Chevy. Because we were only driving about 10 MPH and my car sat lower to the ground, the front of his car humped the back of mine. My back wheel rubbed against his front wheel causing a bumper car skid, stopping us for a brief moment until I had room to pull forward and out from the jaws of his front end.

Fortunately, the traffic gods smiled down on me with an opening in the lane ahead and I accelerated to get away from the maniac. Unfortunately, the driver was pissed and followed close behind.

I ducked in and out of lanes trying to lose him to no avail. The pursuit continued and now the big, angry, driver had his window rolled down and was shouting at me.

"You heet me. Pool ohver."

"Uh, no—YOU hit me!" I screamed back in my most intimidating voice.

"It's NOT a great idea to challenge an incensed brute from Eastern Europe." Jeff said in a calm and serious voice.

"Jeff, I don't have time to argue with you about this, I've got to figure out how to lose this vodka drinking bastard."

Just ahead I saw a sign for the 405 Freeway and sped toward the exit in full panic mode. The ogre followed me bobbing in and out of traffic, still screaming only now the words were in a foreign language, so I had no hope of understanding what he was saying. Probably for the best, since I could make out from the tone that he was furious and ready to engage in Freeway Fight Club.

I steered us safely onto the single lane off-ramp and felt good about my chances of losing him once I made the 200 yards that stood between the wide-open 405 and my shitty Chevy. When I looked back to see how close he was, a new development occurred. There was a third car on the scene. I hadn't noticed it before, but it looked like the tyrant had company, and any friend of an angry car communist is not a friend of mine.

The new *friend* zipped past my car and slammed on the brakes, giving me just enough time to stop my car before crashing into the backend of his Mercedes E class. I quickly (and very instinctually) threw my car into reverse to give myself some distance. Within seconds, the savage was behind me and suddenly *we* were the sauerkraut in their sandwich.

I watched as the enormous gangster exited his car and walked around to his trunk. He was even taller and deadlier than I'd imagined. His shiny, bald head ducked down to search for something in the trunk of his car. Meanwhile, his equally menacing (and huge) brother in arms was getting out of his car.

The barbarian reappeared in my rearview mirror holding a baseball bat. He was approaching my car like the villain in a Hollywood blockbuster. We could hear him mumbling over and over again, "You heet my kar." His buddy was now striding in our direction, too, yelling, "You heet my brutherz kar."

Oh crap! My mind was spinning out of control—I remembered *The Hunt For Red October*, these people know how to exact revenge—even if they were the ones at fault.

Jeff looked at me with terror in his eye and said, "What are we going to do?"

I shifted into drive and scaled up onto the 45-degree concrete dividing wall. My piece of crap Cavalier roared in protest as I cheated around the Mercedes and flew onto the 405 Freeway.

My eyes stayed fixed on the rearview mirror. I knew it would take the tag-team duo some time to get back in their cars and I used my time wisely.

I drove 85 MPH up the 405, testing the limits of both my worn car and our exposed eyes in the G-Force winds. In tears and desperate, I was searching for my next idea. Then a miracle—I saw a California Highway Patrol car sitting in the shoulder lane in the distance. I slowed down and calmly made my way over to the parked police car.

The officer approached my vehicle and asked, "Is everything okay?"

I explained what had just transpired, sparing no detail. During my vivid account of the incident a small grin grew on his face and he nodded, indicating that he understood the volatility of the chase. I didn't really think the story was that amusing, but then again he wasn't the one who almost had his face smashed in.

"So you got away?" he said, challenging my concern.

"Well yes, barely—but what if they find us or report us as a hit a run?" I demanded.

"Not gonna happen," he stated without hesitation. "They were running a scam on you. People do this for a living. They wait until they can corner you and then they try to extort money."

"Really? That's a thing?" I asked in shock.

"Yep. Happens all the time." Then, "Tell you what, I'll take your license and registration and you can have my business card. In the event that they report a hit and run, I'll confirm that you tried to report the *incident*." He took my information and handed me his business card.

"Have a good night and drive safely," he said as he pulled off in his squad car.

Shaken and numb, I pulled away and headed toward our house, making sure to stay on the back roads, while maintaining a lookout for crazy communists. We arrived home safely that evening. Thankfully the officer was correct, the criminals never reported the accident. I learned a valuable lesson: Capitalism inspires fun adventures, but beware of road wars with the Russian Mob.

Only In LA:
Gay Pavilions

Pavilions, which is situated in the heart of Los Angeles' most fabulous and well-maintained area of town, West Hollywood (WeHo if you're a homo-in-the-know), is lovingly referred to as Gay Pavilions.

In this manicured market you can always find fresh fruit shopping for organic produce, overpriced meat (literally), and plenty of spirit(s).

Our story begins when my then *partner*—now husband (thank you, California) and I had to purchase a few necessities for a last minute pool party that we were invited to.

Ordinarily, Jeff and I make a superb team and relish spending a lot of time together. When I'm in a grocery store I like to divide and conquer, mainly because Jeff over-analyzes everything. I'm not complaining—his attention to detail and careful evaluation (of everything) adds a heightened layer of style, refinement, and excellence to our lives. But sometimes you just want to grab a jar of pickles and get the hell out. Where Jeff sees a hundred different options, I see the jar that has the most enticing label and hope for the best.

We were in such a hurry that I easily convinced him that we should split up. I would get the bread, because I'm an expert when it comes to carbohydrates. Thankfully I no longer cared about maintaining a leotard physique in the off chance that the Broadway production of *Cats* called. Jeff could get the wine, because he grew up in Northern California—which automatically makes him a wine *expert.*

I stayed on target while considering my baguette options: Long and thin, or, short and thick? It was a tough decision and I'm a firm believer that there is a time and place for both preferences, but today I decided that the longer loaf would go further with a large group of people.

I weaved through the selection of available men who were pretending to shop for food. Honestly, who do they think they're fooling? Their bodies are proof that the only source of food they consume comes from a protein shake between workouts. I reached the front of the store, deftly avoiding the candy aisle, the magazine stacks, and the deli section (where all of the hot dads hang out), where I saw Jeff already waiting on a line. Given that it was a holiday, the store was unusually busy, and shoppers were extra agitated. I skillfully dodged an unhappy couple bickering about organic vs. non-organic milk—just in time to meet Jeff at the head of a very long line.

The checkout clerk had started scanning Jeff's items as I politely squeezed past the women next in line—a short-statured lady in her late fifties, wearing a balled up cashmere pashmina and mismatched mail order stretch pants, holding a basket full of single serve frozen dinners and a bottle of wine.

"Pardon me, do you mind if I sneak past you to join my friend?" I stated as a way of kindheartedly asking her to get out of the way.

Without waiting for my sentence to conclude she shouted, "Excuse me! There. Is. A. Line. Here. Are you blind?"

"Do you see me holding a white cane?" I snapped back.

"Obviously I know you're not blind. I'm just shocked that you're in such a hurry that you would cut a woman off."

"I'm sorry that you felt like I cut you off. Actually, I acknowledged your presence, by saying excuse me, as I joined my partner—who has been standing in this line waiting for me."

"It doesn't just work like that, you can't have somebody hold your space." She was relentless.

Moments from snapping, I took a deep breath and turned to face her. "Ma'am, I don't understand why you're so offended by me. But I can assure you that we planned on paying together, and my adding a loaf of bread to a transaction that was already in progress will not affect you getting home to your frozen dinner and wine."

"Typical faggot," she muttered under her hideous breath.

I turned around and my tone changed from respectfully sassy to a full-blown Tyra Banks read. "What did you just call me?"

She stood unflinching as I gazed into her beady black troll eyes and didn't utter a word. My head whipped to face the astonished cashier, and before he could offer his thoughts on what just transpired, we heard it again—only this time it was audible enough for our whole line to hear it, "I wish they'd get rid of all you faggots."

I flipped back and challenged her at the top of my lungs, "Did you just call me a faggot, again?"

Then, as if I was delivering a Shakespearian monologue, I used the checkout area as my stage and engaged an audience full of mostly gay men and young hip straight couples. "This woman in aisle four (I pointed at her for dramatic effect) just told me that she wished all faggots were dead. How do you feel about that?"

A small but emphatic crowd gathered to reprimand her to no avail. She continued to utter slurs about gay people while we stood waiting for the bagboy to finish packaging up our groceries.

In a moment of hope I looked at her and asked her for an apology. "Apologize for what? I meant what I said."

I reminded her that she lived in Los Angeles, and that she was shopping in a community where people of all races, religions, and sexual orientations coexist respectfully. My tone was passionate but elevated. As I continued to speak I started to release my emotional frustration.

At this point a mob of appalled onlookers had started to gather around the confrontation, some of who were more incensed than I. The volume and exasperation climaxed and I could see that the woman was feeling overpowered and alarmed.

In an effort to ward off the throng, she threatened to call the police and began fumbling through her handbag searching for her cell phone. Instead, she pulled out an old cardboard camera—the kind you'd see sitting on the table at a wedding reception because your friends wanted you to help them commemorate the day or couldn't afford a photographer—and she began punching the box as if she were using a cell phone.

"Are you pretending to call the police on that camera?"

She was stressed out and confused, but not crazy. She held the instant camera up to her ear and began talking.

"Wow. Okay, well I hope that you will try to be a better person, or at least avoid shopping in gay-friendly areas."

I could tell that she had reached her breaking point. I started to feel sympathy and then remorse. I never intended for the situation to escalate so quickly—all I was really after from her was an apology for using such a vile slur.

Just as I was walking away I noticed that she was wearing a Star of David. I looked at her, referencing the Jewish symbol, and I said to her, "Your people have been discriminated against, persecuted, enslaved, and murdered for thousands of years. I would think that you would have more compassion for a group of people who also suffer from hate crimes."

She was cold in her response. "You people are disgusting, and you made that choice."

I was sad. I was stunned. I was crushed, and I wanted to make her feel as infinitesimal as I did. Looking her straight in the eyes, I asked, "Do you have children?"

She quickly responded, "No."

"Thank God," I replied, "Your hateful heart dies with you."

As the words fell out of my mouth, I felt ashamed. I was so busy driving my message home, that I missed the point all together. Hate is hate, and we were both guilty victims.

Hotel Hook-Up

After splashing cold water on my face, but before turning on the harsh reality of the 3-star hotel lighting at six o'clock in the morning, I do a quick inventory of my face. It is, after all, what I consider my greatest asset. To the outside world I may come across as a hardworking, outgoing, self-confident (albeit slightly narcissistic) man who remains youthful if not in appearance, then certainly by means of my infectious energy. At thirty-eight years old, I stand in judgment of my reflection in the mirror, which confirms that I have spent my entire adult life on the road. The first thought that enters my mind is: It's time for more Botox.

This morning was not unlike any other day on tour. Twenty years of living out of a suitcase teaches you how to devour a fourteen-hour work day and polish it off with a four hour bitchfest over a bottle of wine (okay two) at the hotel bar—still managing to get six hours of sleep before waking up to do it all again.

It was just past six-thirty when I began my daily routine: bedside yoga, a journal entry (usually motivating myself to be positive, while simultaneously making plans to be doing "something" else— ANYTHING else—this time next year), a quick blog post, and then into the shower to wash away the sadness I feel. Rather than performing, I am earning a living critiquing the talent I see on stages across America at one of the country's largest talent competitions.

Once clean and awake thanks to the scalding hot water, I quickly dress, leaving enough time to blow dry my hair, grab a protein bar, and head down to the disgusting continental breakfast, where I meet up with the rest of my colleagues who happily consume the gelatinous oatmeal, four-day-old muffins, and just-add-water orange juice.

Waiting for me with a scandalous story and a devious smile was Judy: blonde, beautiful, talented, and a devious diva. Think Anna Nicole Smith, only alive, intelligent, and from the mid-west (so naturally there's an accent).

"Maaaattthhhewwww, what took you so long? You. Are. Never. Going. To. Guess. What. Happened. Last. Night!"

I sat down eager for something amusing to fixate on for the next ten hours, "Lay it on me—and it better involve handcuffs."

"Ew, no! [Beat] God, I'm not a freak!" She lied. "I fucked Robbie."

"What? I mean don't get me wrong, the man is beautiful and I don't think there's one person in our crew who hasn't commented on the size of his manhood (you can literally see veins through his slacks at the side of his knee) but isn't he a married man with a prescription drug problem?"

"Oh, please Matthew, don't get all judgy. His wife is a total bitch, and they're probably getting a divorce anyway. Don't you want to hear about *it*?"

"Okay, please keep in mind that we are actually talent adjudicators, so technically I get paid to be judgy; and YES. Of course I want you to share every *inch* of the night."

From Judy's reaction I can tell that my play on words was overkill. What Judy doesn't realize is that this was an attempt to find humor in a circumstance that—although gay—I didn't understand. (Contrary to Pat Robertson's theory, not all gay men are sluts.) Judy is more complicated than you'd suspect at first glance. Her heart is big and generous, and so is her sexual appetite. Her drop dead gorgeous façade would imply that everything comes easy to her in life—which might be true—and while she exudes confidence, it only takes one stiff drink during happy hour to uncover that not-so-deep beneath her street smart exterior exists a caged bird with a broken spirit.

While I pretend to listen to Judy revealing the boring backstory leading up to the dirty deed, I wonder to myself: Why do so many of my friends think it's okay to cheat while they're away from their spouses? More importantly, why do they feel so comfortable sharing their indiscretions with me?

"Do I look like someone who would enjoy anal sex?" was the phrase that enticed me to reengage in a two-way conversation.

"Did you have anal sex with Robbie?"

"No! Well *kind of*, but not for long. But NO! I hate it."

"Judy, you can't *kind of* have anal sex—trust me."

"I mean he tried, but I just couldn't; you know what I mean?"

"*Kind of*, but no. I love it." Judy's reaction reveals that I've gone too far, again.

"Judy, you know I adore you, and believe me I know how hard it is to resist temptation, but don't you think it's dangerous to get involved with our pill-popping director, who also happens to be married to one of the clients we work for?"

"I know you're right, I just couldn't stop myself."

Just as Judy confides her lack of willpower, Robbie enters the hotel lobby through the double glass doors still beaming from his free-ride the night before. "Let's go people, I've been waiting in the van for ten minutes—we're going to be late!"

Without taking her eyes off Robbie, Judy leans down to grab her handbag and whispers in my ear, "Just promise me you won't say anything."

"Of course not, but don't worry, his face says it all!"

"Matthew! Stop that, people will hear you."

During one of the elusive fifteen minute bathroom breaks between acts, I walk back into the green room in search of something healthy to snack on, and then (as if waking up from a coma) I remember that this company only believes in supplying food that can be purchased at a gas station on the way to a venue. Doughnuts, bags of chips, waxy chocolates, and bottles of Mountain Dew; obviously stoners are in charge of purchasing the food. I'm convinced they pocket the remainder of the food budget from this multi-million dollar organization for post-show herbal therapy.

After grazing on enough stale Doritos and Dove chocolate candies to tip the scale past my "comfortable touring weight" zone, I decide to take a powernap on the thrift store sofa that terrorizes the room. As I approach the couch, I realize that Judy is crouched behind the backside of the secondhand sofa crying so hard her mascara has become her foundation.

"Jesus, how long have you been there? Did you witness what just went down? Are you okay?" I rambled due to the food shame.

"No, I'm devastated. I just can't believe this is happening."

"What's *happening?*" I was so confused, hours earlier Judy was the most euphoric I'd ever seen her.

"My mom went to pick up my daughter for her soccer practice, and walked in on my husband fucking the nanny!" With that, Judy released a snot-launching sob that made me cringe.

"Shit, I thought that only happened in movies and amongst Hollywood royalty." Not at all understanding the drama, I was trying my best to make light of the situation. Also, less than ten hours ago Judy had her own rendezvous with another lover.

"No, Matthew. It happens to *REAL* people. And it's happening to me! He told my mom that he has wanted a divorce for a long time and didn't know how to tell me."

"Well guess he thought visual aids would be most effective?"

"Stop trying to cheer me up, I'm so pissed I could kill that asshole. I mean, how could he do this to me? I'm fucking gorgeous! I'm smart. I'm funny. I'm so much more interesting than he is..."

"Yes, but you're also sleeping with your boss."

"He doesn't know that!"

I took a deep breath, and then considered for a moment whether to speak the truth or not. "Judy, *you* are all of those shallow adjectives, and so much more. You're also not in love with your husband. If you were, you probably wouldn't need to sleep with Robbie each weekend. Maybe this is an opportunity for you to get out of a dreadful circumstance and discover the woman that is hiding inside you, just dying for the opportunity to break free and soar."

... Is what I really wanted to tell her, but instead I said this: "What a prick. He doesn't even deserve you. Seriously, you are a TEN and he is a negative four. I hope you take him for every last penny, and then leave his ass in the gutter where it belongs. Now, let's get you cleaned up and back in the theater. The sooner we get done with the show, the faster you get to ride the Robbie Express!"

With that, Judy perks up, pulls herself together—like only a former Prom Queen can—and walks arm and arm with me back to the theater. As we pass Robbie standing in the wing waiting to resume with the show, he subtly slaps Judy's ass and winks. I think to myself, "This routine is getting as tired as the cast of the Non-Equity Third National (bus and truck) tour of *Mamma Mia;* I've got to get out of this business."

A Night On
the Golf Cource

Our adventure, like countless others, began late one evening in the middle of *Smalltown*, USA following a mandatory industry function; several of my jaded, overworked and underpaid tour-mates and I chased the pretentious party with enough booze to render us numb.

Traveling across the country on tour is anything but glamorous: 4 a.m. wake-up calls, napping on dirty bus seats from venue to venue, the endless barrage of fast food, wearing the same unwashed clothes for weeks at time, and forget privacy. Fortunately, I found my crew of likeminded people and we bonded over our mutual, unspoken code: collect a check and avoid the drama. These were the same individuals who—as teenagers—hung out under the bleachers in high school smoking Marlboro Red's while drinking Mountain Due; you know, the kids who were already "over it" at sixteen. I never fancied cigarettes or florescent green soda; I did, however, thoroughly appreciate their disregard for rules, fitting in, and most importantly their uncharacteristic insight.

Side note: I proudly stand shoulder to shoulder with my cohorts who smoke at weddings, restaurants, and during intermissions. If there is a cigarette break, I'm beside my cancer-chasing companions ready to fill my lungs with second hand smoke (and most likely die before any of my nicotine-loving friends) all for the sake of freedom, rebellion, and the most intriguing information about *almost* everyone. It's not gossip—it's truth.

As much as I value the reckless behavior I exude when enthralled by these chain-smoking, loveably laidback people, I am an A-Type personality with OCD and control issues. I might splendor in the act of letting go, but NEVER want to get caught doing so. Hence, I openly warn individuals that at the first sign of trouble I will split faster than Kate Moss can rip a butt.

Now back to the story, where our drunken adventure leads us to the middle of a golf course acting how performers in their mid-okay-late-thirties behave while on tour. It's two in the morning. We're too loud and having entirely too much fun divulging our deepest childhood memories via spontaneous improvisational choreography. Out of nowhere, two lustrous searchlights shine above our heads from the police helicopter hovering above us. At the top of my lungs I scream, "everybody run!" simultaneously my friend Lydia shouts, "everybody strike an art installation dance pose". I dove into the nearest shrub. The police helicopter continued past the golf course in hot pursuit of whatever happens in *Smalltown*, USA—I'm positive meth is involved—and I look back to see my friends in a beautiful living art sculpture.

I tumble from the bushes covered in broken twigs and damp leaves, like a dimwitted outcast family member from *Duck Dynasty*. Lydia exclaims with laughter, "you ran!" Everyone in the group begins snorting at my cowardly lion laps and I remind them that I will always run if the possibility of prison presents itself.

We made our way back to the resort swapping scenarios that we would consider worthy of bailing on our friends. Lani swore she'd only ditch her friends if she knew that she could get help for the rest of us; Kevin proclaimed that he would never leave a friend behind, even if it meant serving time; Heather maintained that she would always have her friends back.

One by one, the group declared that they would NEVER leave a solider behind. At last, we're standing outside our friend Irene's room. She had intentionally left the sliding glass patio door to her first floor motel room unlocked to avoid having to return through the main lobby. She slid the door open and like a conga-line at a bar mitzvah we followed in behind. Instantly we realized we had made a huge mistake, the unidentified man in his underwear was our first clue. Before we could get a visual on the female voice coming from the bathroom we hauled ass out of there. Everyone split in a different direction through the courtyard, leaving our disoriented friend standing at the door of the wrong room. It turns out my fearless crew wasn't as brave as they claimed to be moments before. I may have been the first to run, but at least I'm consistent.

That night I learned two things. The first, talk is cheap on tour and, most importantly, always lock and latch your hotel room door. You will thank me later.

Excuse Me, Sir, Your Hair Is Melting

During my senior year of high school, while all of my peers were out partying and having unprotected sex, I sat at home vigorously picking at the acne that had camped out on my face during middle school and continued to fully colonize throughout high school. In between applying venomous amounts of Clearasil and Noxzema to my face, I watched reruns of the Howard Stern Show while plotting out how fabulous my life was going to be once I shed my abominable teenage shell. (I'm still waiting for that moment to actually happen.)

Around the time that my classmates were surely ramping up on the heavy petting I was wrapping up my three hour skincare drills, finalizing the last sentence in my journal, and debating about what to watch next; still very wide awake thanks to the numerous cups of Starbucks coffee I enjoyed throughout the day.

Before I could pop in the VHS tape of *Clueless* (my stand by high school "I don't have a date night" movie) I was sucked into an infomercial promising men false hope of true hair restoral. I was only seventeen at the time, and to my knowledge early male hair loss was not something that ran in my family, so I had no reason to have such an adverse reaction. I sat in dismay watching a parade of follically challenged, yet otherwise handsome men, confess to camera how terrible their life was without hair. Tales of hair inadequacy leading to job failure, sexless relationships, and eating alone sent me into total hysteria.

One by one images of these bald men were replaced with action footage of them playing tennis, giving a speech in a board room, and

193

(my personal favorite) towel drying poolside while shaking off the excess water from their newly fostered fringe. I was both aroused and amused—they had amazing bodies, but upon closer examination I had to ask myself, "Who do they think they're fooling with that fake hairline?"

Even then I was practical about my closeted tendencies. I justified gazing at their half naked bodies as motivation to work out more. Through the TV screen I could feel them accusing me of being gay, so I punished them by finding fault in their hair restoration procedure. Until that moment in my life hair loss wasn't even on my radar. Thankfully the E! Channel had accommodated a new compulsion to preoccupy my sexless, closeted, teenage angst.

Immediately following the ninety-minute infomercial I locked myself into the bathroom that I shared with my younger sister and began self-examining my hairline. Like a monkey grooming his mate, I meticulously combed through each section of my hair trying to count the follicles. I took a tape measure and marked off the distance from my hairline to my eyebrow and recorded it onto a piece of graph paper that I kept in my journal. I stared at myself in the mirror imagining what I would look like bald. I knew it wouldn't be a good look for me

The next morning I woke up with one mission: uncover everything I can about hair loss and make a plan to avoid it at all cost. This would have been a much easier challenge if I was born ten years later and my computer could do more than process words and allow me to engage in early AOL chat rooms with strange men—which I never did—please reference my essay, AOL Chat Room for the truth.

I was at the library researching men's health, which led me to hiding in a corner of the Mystery section, drooling over naked men in textbooks. I achieved a heightened sensation in my pants, but was unable to secure significant insight on understanding the male hair gene. After hours of STUDying, I happened across an article that linked stress, genetics, and too much testosterone to male hair loss. Unhappy with the results I found at the library, I continued my analysis in the magazine section of our local drugstore. After reading several issues of Cosmo, I uncovered that hot oil treatments, daily brushing and prenatal vitamins were all acceptable ways to maintain "luxurious locks".

Never one to waste time, I began my new hair care regimen that evening, which proved to be the perfect spa addition to my skin care torture. It also offered substantiating evidence into the case of my already suspicious sexual orientation.

After a few months of diligent effort, my enthusiasm for hair care began to shift. The prenatal vitamins and hot oil treatments were costly and started getting in the way of my Starbucks addiction.

I'm a practical person; I decided that I might as well enjoy my hair for as long as I had it, and thus started a storm of experimental hairstyles. Over the course of the last four months of my senior year, my hair was: florescent green, Ronald McDonald red, royal blue, circus yellow, purple, and finally jet black.

Two weeks before my graduation day my mom came to me with a simple request, "Would you please dye your hair back to its normal color for graduation?"

Because my mom had always been so supportive of my choices—however colorful they might be—I felt that I owed her one *normal* moment to look back on.

Eager to make my mom happy and to remedy my dry, multi-colored mop—which looked more like a nest that a character from Sesame Street would hatch in—I went to the local drug store the following day. I combed the hair care aisle in search of the perfect graduation day color. After forty minutes of comparing synthetic hair samples against my skin tone, I settled on a box of Natural Instincts Medium Brown. I was sold on the promise of "natural golden highlights", which I thought made the perfect statement: Normal, but not mousy or boring.

Once home, I swiped an old T-shirt from my dad's closet, in order to avoid any unnecessary damage to my cherished designer duds, and locked myself in the bathroom. I tore open the box, mixed the ingredients into the pink plastic bowl and began applying the stinky gelatinous mixture onto my hair with the provided applicator. Never one for instructions, I tossed them into the trash along with the remains of my hair concoction.

I clawed open the King Sized bag of Doritos and began critiquing the images I saw in the US Weekly; both of which were impulse buys at the drug store. By the time I reached the "Who Wore It Best?" section of the magazine, I could feel my scalp tingling.

"Oh good, it's working!" I thought, and I continued to scrutinize celebrities and their poor choices.

As I turned the page on a riveting story, *Getting To Know The Spice Girls*, I felt my forehead ignite with flames that only a New York City fireman (preferably shirtless) could put out. I earmarked the corner of the magazine, which ironically made Posh Spice appear half her size— now *that's* foreshadowing—and set the magazine down on the back of the toilet.

Nothing could prepare me for the tragedy that I faced in the mirror, so gruesome a scene that my neighbors are still talking about the sonic screams they heard.

My dad and sister came running to my aid the second they felt the vibration of my reaction, which penetrated the foundation of our house.

A thunderous knock on the bathroom door preceded, "Son, are you okay?"

No answer.

The knock turned into a fist of panic, "Matthew, are you okay? What's going on? Open up this door!"

"I can't. You won't believe it. I'm ruined."

"Son, I can't help you if you won't let me in."

"Okay, but you have to promise not to be mad."

"I can't promise that, but I promise I will always love you."

"Promise you won't be mad, or I won't open the door."

"This is NOT a negotiation. Open this door now, or I will tear it down." My dad was not bluffing.

I was helpless. The damage had been done and all I could do now was open the door and pray that he might be able to help, or at least assure me that my situation was not as bad as I was making it out to be.

I unlocked the bathroom door and my dad heroically barreled into the bathroom with my sister close in tow. I stood sobbing with handfuls of my melted hair in both hands.

It took a moment for my dad and sister to process what they were seeing, and then in stereo, they exploded with laughter.

"Oh my god! Well, you finally did it—you ruined your perfect hair," my dad snorted.

"Why would you do this?" My sister chimed in with curiosity and judgment.

"This is not funny, my life is over," I barked back.

"Relax. You're not dying—but your hair is," my dad continued to snort.

After the initial comedy of the moment subsided my dad took action.

He turned on the hot water and stuck my head under the sink, washing away the remainder of elixir and golden chunks of oatmeal like mush—which used to be hair.

After several minutes of rinsing, he shut off the water and handed me a towel to dry my hair.

I stared at my reflection in the mirror for several minutes before heading into the living room where my dad and sister awaited to evaluate the severity of my mane-meltdown.

"It's not as bad as I thought it was going to be," my dad said cheerfully.

"I thought you were going to have to shave it all off," my sister added reassuringly.

I knew that they were doing their best to be kind, but my hair was tortured worse than Marcia Clark's—and that was saying a lot at the time. The color was a vague shade of ashy brown with low lights of green and amber. Entire sections were frayed and standing straight up regardless of how much pomade I continued to apply.

After several days of melodramatic pleading, my mom finally caved and took me into her favorite overpriced salon for corrective hair color and keratin treatments. In just under five hours of stripping, processing, and reapplying chemicals, my miracle worker, Stacey, was able to transform my hair back to a natural shade of light brown with notes of red.

Given that thirty percent of my hair had disintegrated into my hands, there was undoubtedly very little Stacey could do when it came to shaping and styling my hair. She was able to cut around the singed sides and top of my hair; but I demanded that she left the back of my hair intact—in a desperate attempt to hold onto whatever hair I had left.

Convinced that Stacey had done everything she could, my mom charged my day of re-beautification onto several different credit cards (which she hid from my dad) and I left the salon looking like a cross between Jonathan Taylor Thomas and Billy Ray Cyrus—it was not my finest look.

The good news is that mom got her wish; I was hardly the only one in my class sporting a mullet on commencement day.

Years later, and still thankfully with a full head of hair, I took a job working with a talent organization that toured across the country hosting talent competitions for young performers. Like most entertainment based companies the roster of employees was eclectic— visualize a group of traveling carnies, but with teeth. Yep, it's exactly what you imagined.

There I was working alongside a merry band of characters, some of whom were incredibly talented and good looking, and others who had boisterous personalities. I found a friend in the latter.

Chad was a large man, less in height and more in girth. I wouldn't call him fat; the word inflated comes to mind. He was no doubt a lady-killer in his time, and while he was still faintly attractive—time, poor eating habits, too much alcohol, and spending half of his life on the road had finally caught up to him. What his skin lacked in hydration, he made up for in charisma, wit, and a well-crafted card trick. Chad was a practiced magician. He reminded me of a former quarterback-turned-defensive coach of an NFL team; if you closed your eyes tight and shook your head from side to side you might be able to sleep with him, once. Did I mention his hairline, yet?

Chad had shake on hair. Not noticeable at first glance, but if you spent more than fifteen minutes in conversation with him your eyes would begin to question the tiny black specks of powder that filled the spaces where strands of hair were absent.

One night after a bonding session where we'd both consumed one too many drinks at the bar, I questioned him about his suspicious hairline. Without hesitation he confessed that he used an upscale sprinkle-on hair product to "fill out" his expeditiously receding hair. No big deal, moving on.

Several weeks later I sat in the audience as Chad, who was also the master of ceremonies for the company, stood on stage announcing the top ten finalists. Normally cool and collected, I noticed that he was sweating heavily. Stage lights are searing enough on their own, but add to it the fact that we were in the sweltering south, and you can imagine the sour state of his suit.

Polished and confident, Chad casually loosened his necktie and continued calling the tiny talents forward to interview them. Each of the contestants stepped up to the microphone and exchanged a brief playful banter before taking their final mark on stage. At last, he had reached the last of the contenders, who was by far the youngest girl in the competition. She approached him like a skittish cat—and always the pro—Chad wasted no time dropping to one knee to make her feel more comfortable. He held the microphone up to her face and asked the young performer the same question he had asked the previous opponents, and she just stared back with an odd look in her eyes.

Chad attempted his usual techniques of engagement to no avail, until finally the talented toddler broke her silence.

She leaned into the microphone with a look of curiosity and horror, and said, "Excuse me sir, your hair is melting."

My heart sank. "I know the feeling!" I thought to myself as I ran my hands through my hair and remembered that unlike Chad's—mine grew back.

We spend so much time obsessing about our appearance. Powders, sprays, wigs, plugs, creams, pills—overpaying for products that promise to transform us into an impossible version of what we see in a magazine or on TV. I'll leave you with this thought: The next time you succumb to the pressure to reach for the next miracle elixir, Google "President Trump's hair", and ask yourself, "Am I really *that* desperate?"

Acting On Adderall

Directing and choreographing children's theater was not at all how I had envisioned my adult life of fame, fortune, and standing reservations at Spago's during the sexless-teenage summer I spent grandstanding at a New York City musical theater camp. Thank the theater gods; I am not afraid of the irony that followed.

I started working with Rebecca out of desperation. Only after I had maxed out all of my credit cards and in between my demanding schedule as an unemployed actor fighting for auditions and my gym workouts, I surrendered to the truth: I needed a job. Any job.

The first clue that I was making a poor choice in my employer came when I sent my résumé and cover letter to the job post, which was advertised on a popular (and reliable) website for entertainment professionals, and the email bounced back. On second glance at the job listing, I noticed a conflict in the spelling of her company's name on the email that was provided. It dawned on me that she must have inadvertently switched the letters in her email. Serves her right for attempting a clever and obscure theatre reference for the title of her company. She CLUEdn't be clever with a pun if her life depended on it.

Starving for a job that would keep me engaged creatively and away from retail ridicule, I tenaciously forwarded the original email to every variation of the cheesy-entertainment-based name I could think of.

Her reply came in the form of a phone call within seconds of receiving my email.

"Hey this is Rebecca Clover. I. AM. SO. IMPRESSED… that you found me! I've had that job listing up for two weeks and I couldn't figure out why no one in LA was interested. We start our first day of rehearsal next week and I was getting desperate!"

"Oh, okay, I understand. I thought maybe this was some kind of test to calculate how resourceful potential job candidates are to get a job in this economy."

Rebecca snorted and followed up with a vulgar laugh-out-loud burst, "Let's meet tomorrow at the Coffee Bean and Tea Leaf on Ventura and Coldwater. I think you're going to be perfect for the job!"

I arrived ten minutes early the following day to further illustrate my exceptional work ethic; director-choreographer types get a bad rap in the industry, and I wanted to make a strong second impression.

Several minutes later I see a crazy woman with faded jeans and a mismatched denim jacket wearing Jackie-O sunglasses and a synthetic wig (that was slightly askew) walking toward my table with a huge smile. We'd locked eyes and there was no looking back now.

Approximately ten steps away from my table, she extended her arms in preparation for a hug. I stood to meet her exuberant embrace and forced my head into an awkward forty-five degree angle, avoiding physical contact with her menacing mane.

We ordered our drinks at the counter and jumped right into conversation. Rebecca is an overbearing, loud, witty woman with a big heart and an enormous passion for theatre. She is also legitimately CRAZY. I'm comfortable with *crazy*—I think it can actually be fun— if administered in small doses. At this point, I was enthralled by the candy-coated spoonful of small talk. After exchanging our mutual love for Hugh Jackman, our disdain for Andy Cohen, and our confusion of Kim Kardashian's talent-to-fame ratio, we discussed brass tacks.

The Facts: Rebecca started a small children's theater company in Sherman Oaks, CA in an effort to provide refuge for the kids who wanted to participate in the prestigious and overpriced afterschool musical theater programs in Los Angeles, but didn't make the cut (or have the discipline required) to perform with the infamous Golden Theater Company, which all of the future stars of tomorrow attended. Also, Rebecca's daughter was only getting ensemble parts at the competitor, so she needed to create a vehicle to give her daughter the star-platform she was born to have. Welcome to LA.

Rebecca was convinced that third, fourth, and fifth graders could spend three hours, twice a week—learning lines, choreography, blocking, and music—while having fun. She also thought you could take a twenty-minute break each week for "play time" because, "at Golden there was too much emphasis spent on training and rehearsals."

I nodded in polite agreement, while my mind was thinking, "This woman is looking for a miracle worker. Thank her for the meeting and move on." Against every ounce of intuition, I took the job.

The *fun* started soon after I arrived home from our first (three hour) production meeting in the form of ten emails in varying tone, some without subject headings and others with only four or five words that had no rhyme or reason. I could already tell that she used her split personality to reel people in—meeting in person to charm them and then hiding behind electronic communication to bully everyone into getting her way.

Everything that we had negotiated at our original meeting was crumbling faster than a lawyer representing Donald Trump.

Oddly enough, considering that Rebecca was a mother, our first battle was fought over appropriate children's content. She wanted our first production to be *Chicago the Musical*. What father doesn't want to see his nine-year-old daughter prancing around stage singing songs about adultery, murder, and prison?

"Yeah, but *Cell Block Tango* would be so exciting."

I begged Rebecca to consider something fun like *Mary Poppins* or *Beauty and The Beast*, but she shot them down in true *Chicago* style.

After running down a list of questionable suggestions including: *Cabaret*: cross-dressers, Nazi's, and strip-clubs; *A Chorus Line*: tits, ass, and homosexual-molestation; *Sweet Charity*: more strippers and sex; and *Rent*, AIDS—do I need to add anything else?—we finally agreed on *Mamma Mia*.

Next step: tackling the daunting script to make it more "rich-industry-kid" friendly. Rebecca suggested that we meet at her favorite Thai restaurant. How did she know I would never turn down anything covered in Green Curry? Our dinner was enchanting. We could talk for hours about celebrities and Broadway, and now that we had polished off the second bottle of Chardonnay, our conversation started to get deep. She confided in me that she missed working with her original director. Of course, I took the bait. Halfway through the conversation, I was sweating—the curry was so spicy that water was pouring down my face as I listened to her reveal just how mentally unstable she was.

I only heard her side of the story, which included blackmail, hidden recording devices, and homeland security. That was all I needed to hear to understand that Rebecca would do anything to get her way. I quickly lightened the mood by suggesting that I was going to drink the bowl full of remaining curry sauce—which was delicious enough that I would have—if not for the fiery heartburn that would erupt as soon as my head hit the pillow.

Ready to wrap this ThaiEYE-opening experience up, I explained that we would need to cut (at least) thirty minutes from our production of *Mamma Mia*. She argued that nobody could be upset with two hours of uninterrupted Australian pop music. I assured her that no matter how adorable children singing and dancing to 70s pop songs might be, no parent or grandparent wants to sit through that.

"The Broadway cast was painful enough," I declared. "I can't imagine children pulling off that (and I use this word loosely) *script* any better."

That's when Rebecca revealed that she fancies herself a writer. "Don't worry, I rewrote the script and injected some humor." Strike THREE! I think… I actually started losing count.

"Rebecca, you can't change the script. The company that you bought the rights from will find out and shut us down."

"Oh, I didn't buy the rights—I don't have that kind of budget. It'll be fine."

At that moment my reservations about taking the job were no doubt comparable to the investor's reactions after standing behind Michael Crawford's Broadway "comeback", *Dance of The Vampires*, which SUCKED, and not in a good way.

Finally convincing her to cut the script, omitting portions of the play that alluded to sex and affairs, we continued with our pre-production work. The time came to hold our auditions and with it, twenty-seven random children who had been rejected by Golden arrived to audition alongside Rebecca's daughter, Kelly, and her entire third grade class (who had all been promised a part).

We had too many people for the musical, but that didn't penetrate Rebecca's mind. She was ready and willing to take them all; even the ones who couldn't sing, dance, or act. Rebecca was first and foremost a businesswoman, and where there's a kid, there's an enrollment fee.

Each child was told to arrive with a prepared monologue and their favorite song to perform; they would learn a short, challenging dance combination at the audition and we would make cuts.

The only thing that was cut that day was my pride. One by one, high-strung, overly confident, heavily medicated, privileged children took center stage reciting poorly memorized speeches they'd no doubt learned while watching a rerun of *iCarly* or whatever popular kids' show was on Nickelodeon or the Disney channel.

I was moments away from losing my mind when I closed my eyes, released my self-esteem, and surrendered to the true description of the job: collecting money from (mostly) neglectful parents who were more desperate for their child to become famous than actually learn a craft. All things considered, the show was well received, securing us the opportunity to further exploit the saturated children's musical theater market.

Rebecca and I hit a clumsy stride by our sixth show. Sure we continued to disagree over script length, content, casting, sets, costumes, the amount of "free time" spent during rehearsal—basically everything. But she (almost) never interfered with my direction or choreography. I considered this a successful working relationship. Plus, I couldn't overlook the fact that she continued to treat me to delicious dinner meetings with plenty of wine (she was smart that way), and it's not like I was booking other work, so I made my peace with the circumstances.

When we sat down to map out our next production, Rebecca pitched me several of her original full-length musicals complete with semi-committed line readings and sloppy marked "arm-ography." The theater gods were on my side that day, because after using a bowl full of non-dairy coffee creamers to represent the blocks that we would stack and move around the stage for "fun levels", I managed to convince her to agree on *Bye Bye Birdie*. Rebecca was a sucker for practical staging that involved being cheap while yielding a high production value.

When casting a children's theater production of *Bye Bye Birdie*, it is imperative that you identify which medications your star might currently be taking, including but not limited to: Xanax, Adderall, Pixie Sticks, or Mountain Due.

After six weeks of very undisciplined blocking, vocal coaching, choreography, and Rebecca-mandated "free time" (which consisted of the children eating fistfuls of sour patch kids and running around the theater) we had finally made it to our tech rehearsals.

I loathed tech week—primarily because it meant spending three hours a day listening to Rebecca complain that nothing was ready. Which would prompt a very matter-of-fact response from me that usually included phrases like: "We would've been ready if we spent more time rehearsing, and less time allowing the children to poison themselves with corn syrup." Or, "Remember when I told you that it was not okay to allow the kids to use rehearsal time for homework?" All of this was useless but like a Bravo Housewife, I was always baited by the drama.

On one particular afternoon we were getting ready to block the closing number, which was always a discouraging task because we had to make sure that every child would have a "stand out" moment in order to deliver on the promises Rebecca made to the deep pockets of nepotistic LA parents in order to secure their "star's" enrollment.

In preparation for blocking, I always have the cast sit in the house and take a role. As I started the roll call, I realized that we were missing Ally, our leading lady—again—and her absence at the previous week's rehearsal was her third official (sixth unofficial) warning. On the first day of every new production, I caution the parents and the young actors that if they miss more than three rehearsals, they may be removed from their role and we will replace them with their understudy.

Knowing that three other kids in the cast would have made a much stronger Kim MacAfee, I was delighted that the under-talented and overly praised princess was yet again absent. Without bias and full of inner elation, I announced that Kelly (Rebecca's daughter) would be covering the role for Ally today. When suddenly a flash of silicone mounds on a stick twirled in late. Without warning—and through overinflated lips—I was being ambushed by an artillery of four-lettered words.

Mrs. Drama-Mama was rushing down the aisle screaming at the top of her lungs, using words that most of these students would surely be using soon enough. I was ready to wash her mouth out with soap, so long as it didn't require me to come in contact with her over-pulled, fully injected face.

I was no stranger to the Helicopter-Hollywood-moms who allowed their nannies to do the disciplining, while they harness their *crazy* for important things like: blackmailing the dean of a private school to assure successful placement for their underachiever, or buying off a casting director to land the lead role in the next Toys-R-Us commercial—but this mom took center stage!

There was no stopping this woman, so I calmly glanced at the group of horrified children in the theater, picked up my bag of "essentials" (which was primarily Advil and earplugs) and exited through the front of the house.

An electrical parade of vibrant obscenities trailed behind, rivaling anything Walt Disney could produce. Rebecca and Mommy-Derangest weaved through the mesmerized onlookers into the parking lot, where I stopped on the parade route, turned around unexpectedly and smiled in her face.

She paused for a moment and then like the former cheerleader she was—continued to moan about how horrible I was. Now that we were safely out of earshot of the children, she sprinkled in a few homophobic slurs in an attempt to get a reaction.

Every bit a cliché of what you'd expect from a children's musical theater director, I snapped my head toward Rebecca and expressed how disappointed I was that she missed every opportunity as a "producer" (and supposed friend) to stand up for me and defuse the situation. Forty; in case you're wondering how many times my head whipped back and forth to drive my message home.

Her money motivated, lame response: "I don't think this is *that* big a deal. Ally is here now, let's just go back inside and get to work."

At last, the reaction that Ally's mom was desperately seeking arrived. Only it was directed at Rebecca. I attacked her lack of professionalism, support, respect, and—to ensure a total knock out—I insulted her fake hair.

No matter how desperate I was for the money, I stormed over to my SUV, revved the engine, carelessly backed out of the parking spot, and popped it into drive. I sped toward the exit, when out of the corner of my eye I saw a familiar plastic flash. This time Ally's mom was running toward the front end of my car. This woman was completely insane!

The monster stage mom jumped onto the hood of my moving car and began crying, "You CAN'T LEAVE, you have to finish what you started! My daughter is the star!"

I flipped the windshield wiper lever to wash her from my car like the insect she was, and when that didn't work I slammed on my breaks. Covered in blue wiper fluid she managed to cling to the car. I rolled down my window and threatened her that she had exactly thirty seconds to remove herself from my vehicle; otherwise she was joining me on a seventy-mile-an-hour rage ride down the 101.

She continued crying, "Please don't leave, I'm begging you. If you quit, my daughter will HATE me."

I took a deep breath, looked her directly in her eyes and said, "She ALREADY does! Now, GET. OFF. MY. CAR!"

I could see her sobbing in my rearview mirror. I was in shock. I couldn't believe what had just transpired. My brain was stumbling to make sense out of a grown woman throwing herself onto a moving vehicle. No self-respecting individual would endure her vile profanity and deplorable behavior, but they certainly wouldn't run her down either.

Within seconds I felt ashamed; I can't believe I said such a hateful thing to a woman who was clearly broken. She had reached a low point or was at least willing to risk bodily harm so that her daughter could remain the star of a children's theater production in Woodland Hills, CA, which might as well be a low point for all of us.

Just before I reached the onramp for the 101 South, I pulled over and decided that I needed to regroup. If I quit, I would be letting down forty-five children who all had similar circumstances. I would be no better than their parents if I abandon them two days before the show. Oh and, Rebecca still owed me for half the contract and my mortgage wasn't going to pay itself.

With less pride than Ally's mother when she ejected herself onto my car, I pulled into the parking lot of the theater and made my way back to the stage. I entered to see Rebecca on stage trying to convince a six-year-old to do a pirouette on the highest platform of our set; I made it back just in time.

In her most assured voice she shouted over her shoulder, "I knew you'd be back." I felt the shame of a heroin addict on my fifth round of rehab. The show must go on, if I want to get a paycheck.

Remarkably, the rehearsal process continued without a hitch, until we came to Ally's big song, "How Lovely To Be A Woman." No matter how you break it down, a third grader will never understand the nuances of a coming of age song, but Ally was convinced (thanks to the coaching that she had received from her neurotic mother) that her choices were strong. As gently as possible, I suggested that rather than singing the song like Britney Spears would (lip sync) at the VMA's, we might want to try a more wholesome approach.

Ally's face went completely blank as she stared directly ahead into the darkness of the house—as if planned—a spotlight captured her face just as it began to contort into a child-like version of Norma Desmond. On cue her monologue began:

"I can't deal with this anymore. I wish I'd never been born with this stupid *problem*. I'm just so angry. I hate that I am so troubled, and I have to take these drugs to calm me down. They make me go crazy, and I don't even know who I am."

Unaware of which "problem" she was referring to, I stood in awe of Ally's ability to so quickly summon up a faux emotional meltdown, which was both hysterical and desperate. All the while I could see her simultaneously assess the reaction from the room—"are they buying it?"

"No," was the unanimous answer. I was not going to drink the punch nor would I let anyone else. We had already suffered through enough theatrical outbursts. I was beginning to think we were on the set of Dynasty. I had to contain the situation before someone was thrown into a fountain.

I took my longest deep-breath of the day, calmly walked up on stage and made direct eye contact with the would-be 80's soap-opera star and gently offered my advice.

"Darling, I know you feel frustrated. I understand how difficult it must be to live with your mom, and I appreciate that you have to take medication for your (mild?) case of Attention-Deficit Disorder, but I can assure you that you are no more special than any other actor in Hollywood. We're *all* nuts. You're going to have to learn how to let the Adderall work for you, instead of against all of us. We're on your side! Now, take a breath, pull yourself together and we'll try it again from the top."

Ally had already reapplied her make-up and chugged a Starbucks Double Shot by the time I reached the tech table in the second row of the theater. My pep talk had convinced her that she belonged among the ranks of Meryl Streep, because that's exactly the caliber of performance she gave the second time through. It was the first honest moment she'd had in the six weeks we'd worked together.

Opening night could not have arrived faster. I was confident that the cast would be dreadfully mediocre in a way that only a parent could appreciate; so my job was done.

Thirty minutes before the performers arrived, my number one stage mom, Linda, was waiting for me at the box office with a bag full of chilled wine—it's show time! She corked the first bottle and began pouring the crisp Chardonnay. Rebecca shot us a look of disapproval, until I produced a third plastic challis and extended the grapevine. I raised my overflowing party cup and toasted to Bob Fosse because the man was a legend who knew his way around women with HUGE personalities—and I wanted to align myself with him—even if our only connection was alcohol.

Halfway through our second Red Solo cup of wine, forty-five stars, each with their *Mama Rose* directly behind, entered the theater toeing the line with make-up cases, costume bags, and Venti cups of overly sugared and extra caffeinated Starbucks in hand. Making sure not to lose my buzz or expose my half-empty glass of wine (Linda can you please fill this cup ASAP?) I calmly directed the cast to their assigned dressing room.

As I'm pointing fingers, I see a large, handsome, important looking man, whom I know is Ally's father. I can only assume that my ass has a fairly large target on it. I tried to duck into the box office ticket booth, but the teenage crew doing the tech on our show was busy making out. I'm happy to know that theater nerds are finally getting some action, but I need to take action or I will be cut! I was now trapped between the box office and a table full of merchandise, artificial snacks, and flowers (damn Rebecca and her addiction to money!). With nowhere to turn, I channeled my inner Paris Hilton, pulled out my iPhone and began fake texting to avoid making eye contact. That didn't work.

The man was relentless and before I could even unlock my home screen, the Tom Brady lookalike was standing directly in front of me.

"Do you think we could have a conversation outside for a moment?"

"I was just getting ready to go backstage and give the actors their pre-show pep-talk. Can it wait until after the show?" At least this way

I might be able to sneak out once the lights go down, and never return again.

"This is very important to me. I promise it won't take long."

I followed the confident man outside to the parking lot, where only hours before his wife had done an impressive Cirque de Soleil dive onto the hood of my car. He stood for a moment, inhaled, looked down at me, extended his hand, and introduced himself as Robert, Ally's father and the husband of a slightly insane, but well-meaning wife.

I was unsure how to react. I wanted to laugh, but that could have been the wine talking; instead I just smiled like a politician and shrugged my shoulders. He was visibly uncomfortable and embarrassed; I was beginning to understand that this was a more regular position for him.

Trying to make light of the fact that his wife had morphed from overworked mommy to Mommy Dearest on crack, I responded in my best "bro-to-bro" tone, "Ah, what are you going to do?"

"I do a lot of apologizing. I love her, but she doesn't always think before she reacts. I'm terribly sorry that she caused such a scene. I heard she threw herself onto your car?... I'm not even sure how to deal with that."

He shook my hand and shared that Ally had not stopped talking about the show. In that moment I felt a deep sympathy for both he, and Ally. I assured him that worse things have happened to me in children's theater (a justified lie) and I thanked him for reaching out.

Linda stepped outside toward the end of the conversation and swooped me up with—you guessed it—another glass of wine (my third, but why are you counting). We casually made our way backstage just in time to find Rebecca threatening the cast, "If you miss an entrance or forget your lines, you will not get the special surprise I have for each of you!"

I pulled her aside. "Rebecca, if you tell them about the surprise (a hideous faux Academy Award trophy—wasted money) it ruins the surprise. *And*, I promise you, these kids *are* going to miss a few entrances!"

Eager to change the vibe in the room, I cheerfully gathered everyone into a large circle and directed them to grab hands. One at a time we went around the circle, in character, sharing our favorite dessert. Kids love dreaming of sugar, and since most of them came in high on it, I figured I'd keep the buzz going. I'm no doctor, but I question the correlation between sugar and Attention-Deficit Disorder.

The house was packed with parents, grandparents, school friends, and innocent friends-of-friends (who were in for a special treat). The stage manager called places and I could feel my heart beat in the lower region of my abdomen—not a great sign.

The house lights dimmed and Kyle, our one-man-band (who could make a keyboard sound like the Boston Symphony Orchestra) hit the first chord and the show was off and running. Remarkably, the opening number didn't suck.

I suddenly thought to myself, "Where did these talented performers come from? And what did they do to my cast?" It's astounding what a little make-up, an overpriced set, and a few stage lights will accomplish. Sure, the direction was stellar, but the smoke and mirrors really sealed the deal.

The highlight of the show ended up being a scene-stealing performance from our *Mae Peterson*. I don't think anyone (including her own parents) expected soft-spoken little Dana with no personality to spring to life like those tiny sponged sea monkeys that emerge when you add water. Give the girl a head mic and just watch her channel her inner-neglected-middle-aged-meddling-mother. I could see the envy in every bead of sweat that fell from Ally's face as she tried to razzle-dazzle around Dana. Her mother was surely cutting herself quietly as she watched the show slip away from her daughter's grasp; Bye, Bye Ally!

I was showered with love from my cast. Starbucks gift cards and bottles of wine from the parents. From Rebecca, I received notes for the next show.

I made my way backstage to thank the crew and Ally's mother was hiding behind the stage left wing. Again, I was trapped like a cockroach. She was holding an expensive bottle of champagne and held her arms out open wide, "We did it!"

RAID a minute, "We"? She might be able to convince the soccer moms in her social circle that she's a likeable person, but her bubbly act was not working on me. I graciously accepted the Perrier Jouet and walked away.

My time with Rebecca had clearly run its course. I was ready to take a bow but it was hard for me to walk away from the money. I'm the type of person who can't just burn a bridge. I have to torch the valley and villages that surround it, in order to move on. I wasn't planning on stealing the show by making a scene on closing night, but that's exactly what happened—and my performance was definitely worthy of the shitty plastic statue that Rebecca presented me with instead of a bonus check.

No surprise there, I'm unsure of why I held such high expectations for Rebecca. Suddenly, flashes of our past encounters plagued my head...

.... The first big blowout I had with Rebecca was during an early production of *Grease*—when she thought it was important to keep the lyrics, "You know that I ain't bragging, she's a real pussy wagon" in the show—the average age of our cast was nine.

When we produced *The Sound of Music*, she insisted, regardless of her own faith (and the objection of most of the parents), that we include the swastika on all of the "German Nazi" costumes.

One time during a blocking rehearsal for a predominately Latin based show choir at an area high school, she declared to the cast that my choreography looked too "sissy" and that we needed to "macho it up a bit". The teenaged boys called me *joto* for the rest of the semester.

After a rehearsal in the basement of a Christian community center, she told me that I was too hard on the kids during the choreography classes because I gave them corrections, and if I didn't change my tone she would replace me. My tone? I laughed in her face and walked outside toward my car. She followed me, screaming at the top of her lungs. I told her she was a lunatic and she should start looking for my replacement immediately. We engaged in a fifteen-minute "Fuck you!" exchange, matching each other tone-for-tone. Her ten-year-old daughter was our mediator.

When her Macintosh desktop computer crashed, I escorted her to the Genius Bar at the Westfield Mall in Sherman Oaks where she repeatedly berated the not-so-genius employee who didn't ask her if she'd backed up her hard drive before he wiped it. I spent the following two days reinstalling her software. As a thanks, she accused me of "taking my sweet time". I didn't feel sorry about deleting her "original ideas" folder off her hard drive.

And once, at a Mexican restaurant, she answered her phone in the middle of our conversation. She proceeded to talk to the mystery caller for thirty-five minutes; when I politely asked her to rejoin our dinner meeting; she threw a tortilla chip covered in guacamole at me...

The wine-induced recollection in my head ended as Rebecca approached a group of parents sharing their praise.

With a pat on the back and a snarky quip she exclaimed, "Well, you're no Bob Fosse."

"And you're no Cander and Ebe!" I shot back without missing a beat.

"What's that supposed to mean?"

"It means that you're a shitty writer and piss-poor producer who makes false promises to parents for the sake of money. The only thing less convincing than that abominable synthetic wig you wear, is the transparent act that you care for anyone other than yourself. Thankfully, you taught me several life lessons: Think twice before responding to an online ad, avoid mixing children's theater and sugar, always trust your initial instincts, and NEVER convince yourself that you can tame a hairless shrew."

Match lit. Bridge burned. End Scene.

Fighter

I was sitting in an oversized reclining lounge chair similar to the ones you see in bargain furniture warehouse stores. Not at all comfortable. I watched my grown sister slowly raise half a spoonful of applesauce to her mouth and miss her lips by an inch. The frustration in her eyes spoke louder than the dialogue that she scrambled to compose in reaction to the watchful pry from our family, physical therapist, and nurses. One week away from her thirty-fifth birthday and she was relearning how to do everything. Mundane activities that healthy adults take for granted, like brushing her hair, walking, and going to the bathroom were Mount Everest level expeditions.

I was too young to remember what it was like watching my baby sister learn to walk the first time around; now I'm exceedingly aware of her first steps toward recovery. Observing her clumsily transfer weight from foot to foot was similar to the summer I spent at Boy Scout camp where I witnessed a foal take its first steps. The tiny legs are long and strong, but they haven't mastered the exchange of energy and thus become unstable and less graceful than you'd expect from a full-grown horse. My sister's mind tells her she should be able to stand up from her wheelchair and walk to the bathroom, the only problem is she hasn't quite conquered the art of balance.

Even as a toddler, I recognized that my sister was an indomitable force that I would spend a lifetime safeguarding. At four years old I watched my diaper-clad sibling crawl toward the edge of the staircase, which led to an unfinished cement basement. My sister, Shiree, was scaling the wooden "safety" railing the way Tom Cruise effortlessly

215

shimmies across a towering rooftop in pursuit of a bad guy in one of his epic and entertaining blockbuster movies. Shrieking at the top of my lungs for help, I reached for the gate attached to the staircase banister just as it became unhinged. Together, Shiree and I toppled down the skyscraper of stairs, landing unscathed in a neglected basket of laundry.

Long before helicopter parenting became the key to ruining any chance of a child's ability to navigate the world on their own, our parents—who both worked full-time jobs—knew it was perfectly acceptable to entrust me with the awesome responsibility of co-parenting my kid sister. We spent a lot of our childhood looking out for one another. Whether on the playground, before and after daycare, or in dance class we formed a tribe of two, guarding each other against house fires, bullies, and bossy adults.

Like most siblings, we spent the better part of our childhood fighting over ownership of the armrest in the back seat of my parents' car; still when it came down to interference from an outsider, we always joined forces. I had a built-in best friend who enjoyed all of the same activities as I did. Shiree was a total tomboy, so it was never hard to convince her to help me build a fort, swing from a tree rope into a muddy pond, or collect creatures for our multi-purpose glass aquarium; at any given time you might find snails, lizards, or hermit crabs. I was a massive mama's boy; thankfully mi amigo equally enjoyed playing with Barbie Dolls, Fisher-Price Playsets, and Cabbage Patch Kids as much as I did, too. My sister was the perfect disguise for my obsession with "girl" toys (and hot boys). It makes sense now. I was a young boy with a big personality, a short fuse, and really in touch with my emotions. Shiree was a young girl with a big personality, a short fuse, and really in touch with *my* emotions.

Throughout my entire fifth grade year, Shiree and I would rush home after school and pop in the VHS tape of *Dirty Dancing* (which was rated R and entirely forbidden by my parents). We both loved the dance sequences and spent hours practising the ballroom steps. Without fail, every time we reached the sex scene—just as Patrick Swayze was rolling his gorgeous naked body out of bed—I would hit the pause button on the machine and my sister would gaze at his firm ass in awe. It was a nice reward for all of our hard work and utterly indisputable that I fancied Patrick's ballet-toned buns as much as she did.

In middle school, Shiree wasn't afraid to strike up conversation with boys or even join a game that the boys were playing, which segregated her from the norm. Girls at that age can be devastatingly mean to one another and my sister's friends were no exception. They were jealous of the attention my sister received from the boys in her class.

Boys are no dreamy romantic lakeside picnic at that age either. When the rest of the man-boys in my class were busy growing body hair and discovering their enlarging manhood, I was occupied suppressing my creative flair and zealously masking my lack of excitement about the WWF, Nintendo, or rollerblading. The guys in my class would hurl endless derogatory insults and make fun of my appearance, fashion choices, after school activities, and studious work ethic. Subsequently my sister and I battled the trials of adolescence as allies.

When we reached high school our hormones were raging and so were our tempers—thanks dad! We spent a lot of time bickering with each other to disguise the pain that we were subjected to at school. Making matters worse, our parents were going through a divorce that was utterly unexpected. Rather than being there to support one another—as we had throughout our childhood—we grew angry and brutish towards each other. Siblings fight, there's no question about that, but Shiree and I found an impressive level of resentment and we didn't hold back from wringing each other's necks over the silliest squabbles. We had been through a lot of torment, turmoil, and triumphs together, so it was hard for me to lose my best friend when I really needed her most.

Typical of most teenagers, I never expressed my true feelings to her, opting instead to lob insults, which echoed the terrible things that her enemies at school attacked her with. She retaliated with the same vicious put-downs that I faced from my Fag-hater fan club, further validating the shame in my head.

By my senior year of high school, our word-violence and dramatic feud got MTV real!... *The Real World: San Francisco (a la* Puck and Pedro), to be exact. Which was our favorite TV show at the time and the only thing we still had in common. Honestly, do you remember the outrageous acts of drunken hook-ups that happened on that show?

One afternoon my sister and I were splitting hairs over something so unimportant I couldn't even recall the issue if you offered me an Academy Award® winning role in a Wes Anderson film. The aftermath of our fight, however, is every bit as clear as the time I walked into an airport bathroom where an incredibly obese man stood buck-naked drying his tighty-whities under a Dyson hand dryer—some things you just can't forget.

After twenty minutes of screaming back and forth, I decided to raise the stakes. Threatening her to concede, or I would tell our dad that she was dating a 24-year-old MAN. Without hesitation she roared back with an energy that was disavowing and certain. "If. You. Do. That. [LONG DRAMATIC PAUSE] I'll tell everyone that you're GAY!"

The room went silent.

It was the first time that anyone in my family had actually confronted me with those words. My sister was the only person in my life who *really* knew me. Until this moment, she had always sheltered me from having to deal with what must have been obvious to everyone.

The magnitude of my sister's accusation caused my ears to ring. My entire face flushed and my hands and feet went numb. My heart felt like it was filling with cement and rapidly sinking to the pit of my stomach causing a big empty void. I remember feeling the tears on my cheek but don't remember crying. Before I could even form a defense against the prosecution, my sister had already responded for me, by throwing out the trial.

She extended her arms, pulled me in close, and held me tight in a loyal embrace until I stopped crying. Rare for Shiree, she had always been more of a light-hug, pat-twice on the back, and release kind of girl. Once I was breathing without gasps for air, she sat down next to me and apologized. She calmly communicated how much she loved me and promised me that she would never say something like that again. Knowingly conspiring to keep my dark secret camouflaged just as she had done, without my knowledge, throughout our childhood.

I abandoned Shiree three months later to begin *my* life in Chicago.

As a child, a weak immune system and severe urinary tract infections detained my sister to an exam room—a lot. In middle school she suffered chronic strep throat and tonsillitis, which kept her in the hospital more than in homeroom, and just after she graduated high school she had an emergency appendectomy. Shiree visited the hospital as much as most teenagers update their profile picture on Instagram.

My family likes to keep things from me. I don't think they do it on purpose, I just think it's one of those out of sight out of mind kind of things. "Didn't I tell you your childhood dog died? No? I could have sworn I did. Well anyway… yes, I'm sorry, but Elway is dead."

So when, nine months into her sublimely suited career as a police officer—a job that she had invested two years in school working towards—she called me out of the blue and said, "Matt, I have to tell you something, but I don't want you to worry. I'm going to be FINE…" I immediately lost my shit.

Tears gushed down my face as I listened to her explain that in between dealing with small town crime and corrupted city officials, she had discovered a small lump on her neck. She waited to reach out until her doctor confirmed that it was cancer. Hodgkin's Lymphoma stage IIB, to be precise.

"It's the good kind." My sister shared like she'd won the lottery.

"Is there a good kind of cancer?"

"Well, no. But, the doctor said that if you're going to get cancer, this is the good kind. Most people don't survive non-Hodgkin's lymphoma."

The conversation was not reassuring. Adding insult to injury, she was fired from her job as a cop on a technicality. Her "probation" period was ending and rather than supporting her in a time of need, they dumped her like a DA dumps evidence in a murder trial. Shiree endured with courage, asserting that she would fight and survive cancer.

Many rounds of chemotherapy, a succession of radiation treatments, and plenty of painfully repulsive days over the course of a six-month period left my sister exhausted, but cancer free. On a routine follow up two years into her remission, her doctor detected rheumatoid arthritis. This oppressive disease was most likely the origin of her body's lifelong assault against health, which eventually lead to her cancer and firmly secured an endless series of drug infusions to combat the complications of RA.

To her great fortune and the surprise of many medical professionals and concerned family members, my sister gave birth to a beautiful, healthy baby girl just five years after crushing cancer.

Ten years cancer free and five years after Shiree gave birth to my adorable niece, Kellyn, I was wrapping up a job in Los Angeles and received a troublesome phone call from my mom. A volley of follow-up text messages and voicemails came from my dad, my cousin, and two of Shiree's best friends hammering the harsh facts. Shiree had been admitted directly into the ICU due to a sustained temperature of 104.5 degrees and an un-diagnosed illness.

I flew to Colorado to be with my sister on the first flight available.

Once at the hospital, my family greeted me with a look of defeated desperation. Even my father, the most faithful man I know, looked like he'd lost all conviction. Could she really be that bad? Before entering her quarantined room, I was instructed to put on gloves, a gown, and a mask because the doctors had not ruled out a number of airborne viruses that may have rendered my sister catatonic.

Suited in my paper armor, I found myself at her bedside and instantly gushing. Looking down into her exaggerated and expressive eyes that were usually full of joyous vibrancy, I saw no trace of her inner light. I knew that I would stay by her side until she made a full recovery and returned home to her family. Not out of guilt or for praise, but because she needed me to fight for her as much as I depended on her throughout childhood.

The father of her darling daughter was sporadic, unstable, and unwilling to face his fear of inadequacy—or stop drinking long enough—to stand beside her failing body.

Three days, countless tests, and several specialists later, doctors finally concluded that a mosquito carrying the West Niles Virus was the cause of my sister's condition. Most people infected experienced little to no symptoms. Some may develop flu-like symptoms that will eventually go away without treatment. Then, according to her doctor, there are those including infants, the elderly, and people with weak immune systems who fall into a "less than 1% category". These "lucky" people may develop a serious, sometimes fatal, neurologic illness.

After surmounting so many setbacks already in her life, I was disheartened that her spunky disposition was missing along with her toothbrush and toothpaste—hospital halitosis is intense. Granted she'd been laid up in a semi-conscious state for a week, but she's always been such a resilient, determined firecracker. I thought for sure her tenacity would endure. Instead, she masked sadness with a subtle grin and passed off pain with a shrug of her shoulders. What's worse, her *baby daddy* (he hates when I use that phrase to define him) was off gallivanting on vacation in the mountains, binge-drinking to cover up *this* agonizing inconvenience. Meanwhile, my sister and their daughter needed his reassurance, even if it was only in the form of his body—bedside.

Two weeks passed as Shiree slowly emerged from a non-responsive, bedridden patient into the beginning stages of a functioning human. I pushed her to surrender to the daily occupational, physical, and speech therapy despite the agony and fatigue she faced just trying to lift her arms above her head.

Day in and day out I documented which drugs the doctors were pushing, supervised her vitals, and maintained as much conversation as possible to keep her progress on track. I was an annoying cheerleader encouraging her to "Go. Fight. Win!" while watching her exasperation as she tried to pronounce the letter "s" for the speech therapist or stand up and walk along the parallel bars for the occupational therapist. The enormity of the everyday tasks through my sister's body betrayal promoted in me an overly emotional, completely overwhelmed, and utterly sleep deprived state of mind.

I filled my days wheeling her around the rehabilitation center from one doctor to another. Each morning I woke up early to get myself dressed and ready to help her face the day. We started the mornings with a trip to the bathroom, which included transferring her from her bed to the wheelchair and then rolling her into the facility. I would ring for a nurse to take over once she told me that she had finished.

My sister is a very private person, so these exchanges were difficult in the beginning. Three weeks in, I made peace with my temporary, uncomfortable living situation; Shiree accepted that I would have to act as her personal caregiver. A job that you're not prepared for as a sibling, but like a vegan who enters a hot dog eating contest for a million dollar prize, somehow you rise to the occasion.

Our mom and dad would arrive every morning around breakfast and stay through the early evening. As a family we would take turns pushing and praising her small victories. We fell asleep to reruns of *The Golden Girls*, just like we did every Saturday night during our childhood. I'd stare out and daydream about our childhood as she lay sleeping. It was satisfying having our mom and dad together, even under the circumstances. I was enamored with how thoughtfully my mom and dad and their spouses united with me to provide my sister around the clock care, love, support, financial stability, and laughter.

I was caught off guard one morning when I woke up to my sister's question.

"Matt. Where's James?" James is the fictitious name of her "common-law-husband". I changed his name so that my magnificent niece would never have to see his name in writing.

I debated lying. Since she'd been admitted into the rehabilitation center, James had visited less than five times. He was selfish and decided to drown his sorrows in cases of beer and posting desperate social media pleas for attention. I found it remarkable that this *Duck Dynasty*, homophobic, and perpetually unemployed deadbeat—whose favorite pastime was hunting and skinning deer while inebriated—couldn't bear the burden of guarding his family when they needed him the most. And *I'm* the sissy?

I eased into the conversation with my sister slowly. The nurses warned us that it was natural for patients to suffer from depression during stages of rehab, but there was more beneath the surface. I had my diving gear on and I was ready for a deep-sea expedition.

I took a deep breath and replied, "James went to Beaver Creek."

Her eyes slowly began to squint and her face became grossly contorted; her speech therapist would have been proud of her for exercising her facial expressions.

"No, he said he was taking Kellyn camping for the night!" She forced out the words, already realizing he'd lied to her.

"Yes, I think that was the original plan, but he ended up meeting up with the rest of the family. I think seeing you like this was too much for him. He said that his mood was making Kellyn sad and they needed to get away."

"Oh," she muttered—then, "He's weak. Men are weak. Sorry, no offense."

I sympathized with her and offered my apology.

"I don't get it. Wasn't he the one who brought me into the ICU? You'd think he'd want to be here with me?"

In order to reduce the blow and keep the peace with my niece's father, I stressed how overwhelmed he was. I went on to make excuses for him and then reminded her that he had come to visit her the day before.

"Yeah, for like five minutes."

I witnessed my sister absorb the information with a guttural sadness. The man whom she had stood by through multiple "setbacks" (I'd love to rip into his sordid past but I will spare my sister and niece the embarrassment) ditched my sister. He exploited my niece in an effort to manipulate the situation, all to spend a few nights in a magical mountain town with my extended family, who opted to take a previously scheduled (and prepaid) vacation, rather than *deal* with my sister's condition.

It never occurred to James that he should seek help, stop drinking, clear his mind, and step up to the plate. Instead, he got passed-out-drunk every night and relied on the generosity of others to cook, clean, and comfort Kellyn while my sister suffered in silence.

By the end of the fourth week, Shiree and I had mastered the ins and outs of rehabilitation. She was on her way to a full recovery. Her speech was clear, and though it had a different timber from how she usually spoke, I was elated that she didn't seem to suffer any permanent damage. We were laughing regularly and confiding in one another about life, love, and our unmanifested dreams. I felt the impact of how much I'd missed my sister and I cherished that I had the flexibility in my career to be by her side.

One evening while watching reruns of *Law & Order*, my sister's favorite show, she revealed to my dad and me that she had not had a bowel movement in two days. From my own personal experience (please reference *Shit Happens*), I knew that this was not a pleasant feeling. My dad, who was no stranger to his children's BOWEL habits, suggested that I contact the nurse.

Moments later, our favorite nurse, Troxanna, appeared with a suppository and informed us that her blockage could cause severe complications if we didn't act fast. My sister was less than pleased about what was about to happen, but this *shit* was serious. My dad and I left the room and Troxanna went to work. Three minutes later we were invited back into the room and told that it would probably be a few hours before it would have an effect. Dad wasted no time asking, "Was that a pleasant experience?"

She responded, "The going in part wasn't, but this next part might be!"

Suddenly Shiree's face went white and she grabbed the rails of her hospital bed. Squeezing her butt cheeks she shouted, "I gotta go. NOW!" She reached for the red cord to call the nurse. Dad and I started laughing so hard we nearly soiled our own pants.

Troxanna and the night nurse came running past us with gloves and a bucket; we took that as our cue to take a trip to the kitchen for a cup of coffee. Not long after her explosive episode, her doctors (and the insurance company) decided that she had reached an adequate level of progress, and Shiree was released from rehab to continue recovery at home.

We survived the challenges of childhood, withstood the test of teenage hormones, and—thanks to a near-death experience—we rekindled our connection as best friends. The circumstances were traumatic, but the bonding was brilliant. I rediscovered my sister as the unconditionally loyal and loving friend, warrior mother, and fearless fighter who refused to settle for anything other than a full recovery.

Three years have transpired since my sister fell ill. To the untrained eye, it appears as though Shiree is back to her old feisty self. Closer inspection from "Dr. Brother" reveals subtle differences in the way she laughs, communicates, or processes information. Still, she shocked her doctors, friends, and several family members by standing up out of the wheelchair that they were positive she would grow old in.

James is lost in addiction. He slunk away from Shiree last year, offering no financial or emotional support, leaving her to maneuver through life, while nurturing a confident, intelligent, and well-adjusted daughter. Like a Sherpa, she faces each mountain with an adventurous spirit and brave tenacity. Abandoned by her insurance provider, abandoned by James, and repeatedly abandoned by her health, she traverses up the impossibly difficult terrain. With every step, switchback, and setback she unearths an irrepressible, enlightened version of herself. My sister's valiant expedition through life has taught me the most influential lesson thus far: No matter the hurdle, never abandon who you are.

Gram

I discovered death in second grade after a classmate left school early because his grandmother passed away. Prior to that, it had never occurred to me that people didn't stay on this earth forever. When I got home I questioned my parents about the process and my dad explained that once our life ends here, we join in heaven with all of the people that have gone before us. I was unsatisfied with his answer and I did not look forward to saying goodbye to anyone— least of all my family.

The following weekend my grandma and grandpa were visiting us and I cornered my grandma on the couch to gain her perspective. I remember sitting on her lap caressing the soft skin on her face and breathing in the sweet smell of Dove soap and perfume as she gently and lovingly explained that we all have a purpose on earth, and that once we meet our purpose, God brings us to heaven to continue helping him.

I looked up at my grandma and said, "Grandma, when you die, I'll kill myself so that I can be with you there."

She was so calm and wise in her response. "Promise me that you will never do that. No matter how difficult your life gets or how much you miss me, or anyone that you love, you have to stay here and carry on their memory until it's your time. Can you remember that?"

I was devastated at the thought of living without my grandma, but even at eight years old, I understood how important this was to my gram, and so I promised her that I would remember her conversation.

With a pure and nurturing demeanor, Gram could inject herself into any circumstance and provide a unique and effective solution. Her smile was so magnanimous, she left every room in brighter spirits than when she entered and taught me to do the same, which was her trademark for everything in life. "Always leave things better than how you found them."

I consulted her above anyone else in matters of great importance for the simple fact that she listened to me, but never told me what to do. She talked me through all of the possible outcomes that accompanied my scenario and how I might react to them.

When I was in middle school and I had to choose between attending a school dance or a rehearsal for a play that I had signed up for, not understanding the time conflict. She walked me through a list of pros and cons, leading me to make the "right" choice and further developed my problem solving skills.

I was an intense kid who worried a lot, obsessed a lot, and spent a lot of time overachieving. When most of my loved ones and role models would advise me to "relax", my grandma would celebrate my tenacity, guiding me toward outlets, which required using both sides of my brain. She wrote poetry and shared her creative passion with me, pointing me toward writing my feelings down in a journal—which evolved into entering creative writing contests.

During my last year of high school I volunteered alongside her in a nursing home. I watched as she patiently listened to the same stories over and over again. Every time finding a thoughtful new response, validating these under-visited senior citizens. She led group activities and maneuvered through unpleasant interactions with a contagious laughter that stung even the toughest of curmudgeons.

She worked a fulltime job, while taking care of my grandpa's declining health, cultivating her creative hobbies, attending church, holding seats on the Library Board and the Chamber of Commerce, all while finding time to serve the Democratic party.

During the 2000 Presidential Election, my gram and I stayed up late celebrating the victory of President-elect Al Gore only to wake up the following morning and realize that George W. Bush was actually the next President-elect. Rather than freaking out, like I did, she smiled and said, "God keeps us guessing for a reason."

Jeff and I had been living together for many years. We had successfully moved across the country together, and took many trips to Colorado to visit my family; still I waited much longer than I should have to tell my grandma I was gay. Not from fear of her reaction; I knew my gram's love was endless. She was also perceptive and (I'm sure) keenly aware of our relationship; but because she was active in so many clubs and church related organizations, I never wanted to vocalize it, and risk putting her in an uncomfortable position with her friends.

Jeff and I were featured in a national gay magazine highlighting a series of viral pop culture parodies that we created—some in which we portrayed women in drag a la Bosom Buddies—and I decided it was the perfect time to come out to her. I left a copy of the *Instinct Magazine* article next to her morning cup of tea and escaped the house with my dad for an emergency dose of Starbucks. I chugged my Frappacino faster than usual, anxious to return to my grandma for her reaction. She was sitting in her chair giggling when I walked through the back door.

"What do you think?" I asked.

"I think it's pretty neat! You boys are in a magazine for your work!"

"Yes, but what about the *other* part?

"You mean, you and Jeff? Well I love you guys, of course!"

"I know that, but I guess I was worried that your friends might not be so nice to you if they knew…"

"Who cares about what they think? Matt, I will always love you no matter what. Remember: never pay any attention to what people say about you, good or bad. They don't know what it's like to walk in your shoes any more than you do theirs. Just focus on setting the best example you can in your life and let your actions speak louder than your words."

My grandma was in her early seventies when she was officially diagnosed with Parkinson's Disease. Unofficially, I knew a few years earlier. Not in a mystical psychic kind of way; instead I found out on a quick trip to Colorado to visit my family.

After a fun game of dominoes with my grandparents, gram wanted to show me something in their bedroom. As I walked with her through the living room towards their room, I watched my grandma lose her footing and shuffle back a little bit. When I asked her if she was okay, she shrugged it off, noting, "Sometimes you lose your balance when you get older."

As a dancer, I understood what it looks and feels like to lose your balance—this was more than that—I knew it, and I know she knew it, too.

The following morning I brought this to the attention of my dad and my sister, both of whom had also recognized little "moments" similar to the one I witnessed.

"How long has this been going on for?" I demanded from my dad.

"It's been a few months."

"Have you confronted her?"

"Of course I have. She doesn't want to deal with it."

"What does that mean dad? Clearly, something is wrong, she needs to go to the doctor."

"She doesn't want to. She's focused on getting grandpa healthy right now."

"Well we have to do something. What do you think it is?"

"I think she might have Parkinson's Disease. She's got the 'Parkinson's shuffle.'"

I was crying before my dad even finished the sentence. The moment that I had anticipated with dread since second grade was upon us, and it felt too soon. I was desperate to get to the bottom of my grandma's condition. We spent the day preparing spaghetti and meatballs for our Sunday dinner; a tradition that has been a part of my life since birth and continued—without me—after I'd departed to the land of selfishness AKA show business. Capitalizing on the family gathering, I thought that we could unite and convince my grandma to go see a doctor.

I finished my second plate of pasta with extra sauce and (at least) two loaves of Italian bread and butter, which I dipped in even more sauce and the leftover ranch dressing in my wooden salad bowl. Very Italian—I was headed into an emotional warzone unannounced and without alcohol—I needed fuel to initiate the intervention.

"Gram, I've only been visiting for a few days, but I've noticed that you're not getting around like you used to and your hands don't seem as steady either."

With a playful chuckle she shrugged, "I'm getting older, Mattski (a nickname that my grandma and grandpa would use), I'm not going to stay beautiful forever."

Clearly, I had inherited my ability to disarm and distract via lighthearted self-deprecation from my grandmother.

"No gram, I think it's more than that. Have you been to the doctor recently?"

"Yep. He said I'm fit as a fiddle."

"Really? Did you discuss your *shaking* and *shuffling?*" I used these key words to expose that we knew she was keeping something from us.

"Maaaatttt, don't you worry about me; I'm fine."

"Gram, everyone *here* might let you get away with that answer, but I want to know what's going on. You're only seventy-three, that's too young not to take action, for whatever your situation may be."

My grandma rarely raised her voice—never at me—and I could see that she was becoming exasperated. "Matt, I don't want to discuss this. I'll be okay. We have to focus on getting grandpa healthy first, then I promise I'll go to the doctor and prove to you that I'm healthy."

I decided to press the issue further despite the shift in her tone. I wasn't ready to accept her concession to the undiagnosed but totally obvious illness.

"Gram, how can you be here to see grandpa through his battle with cancer if you can't even take care of yourself?"

She snapped, "Matt, I don't want to talk about this anymore. Now, who wants dessert?"

On the last day of my visit home, my grandma had reconsidered my relentless plea. She informed me that she would go to the doctor to figure out what was going on. I was relieved and hopeful that medicine would save my grandma and buy me more time with her.

In the weeks following that exchange, her doctor confirmed that she had Parkinson's Disease, and by his *best* guess-timate, she had probably been living with the disease for over a year. If diagnosed sooner, we might have been able to prolong the inescapable for several years—but *we* didn't catch it in time and now all we could do was play catch up.

She started off on a treatment plan, which we soon realized was not a science. Her doctor switched her pills out faster than Anna Wintour changes moods during a power meeting, until they finally found something that she seemed to respond to.

During the first two years of medical treatment my grandma's health seemed to return to "normal". She was more alert, no longer shuffling along as she walked, her speech was clear again, and her peppy energy returned. It had been years since she could write anything that didn't look like a toddler scribbling with a Crayon, so my spirits and faith were lifted when I received a hand written note from her. "Never too old!" Three simple words written clearly, reminding me that I'm never too old to learn something new, never too old to follow my dreams, never too old to come out of the closet. Even in the midst of dealing with my grandfather's rapidly spreading cancer and her own advancing disease, she found time to support me. At thirty-four-years-old, my grandma was still my best friend and undoubtedly receives the Executive Producer credit in my life's movie.

I've never met two people more in love than my grandparents. They continued to find happiness and laughter in the everyday moments throughout their battles with illness.

I watched them exchange flirtatious glances with one another up until the very end, when my grandpa's body could no longer endure; he passed shortly after their 54th wedding anniversary. I assumed his role as my grandma's daily reminder to take her Parkinson's medication. Five times a day I called my grandma to make sure she stayed on schedule. It was a duty that I was happy to do.

No matter where I was or what I was doing, when my iPhone alarm went off, I interrupted the task at hand and called my grandma. If I was in the middle of a rehearsal, I called her; at a movie, I stepped outside and called her; washing dishes, I called her; at the gym, I called her. On the occasions that I knew I'd be detained—on an airplane or performing on stage—I arranged for a friend or family member to call on my behalf.

*   *   *

Agitated and nervous, I paced in front of a crowded movie theater in Los Angeles tapping my fingers against the backside of my iPhone which was glued to my ear counting the number of rings—4, 5, 6, 7... come on gram, please PICK. UP. THE—finally: "Hi Matt. I'm here. I'm here! I took my pills and the girls say hi!"

In the background I can hear a group of rowdy silver-haired sorority sisters laughing and shouting, "Hi Matt! We told your grandma it was time to take her pills. We're getting her drunk! [Laughter breaks out] You're a good grandson."

"Okay gram, I'm glad you took your pills. I'm getting ready to watch a movie with Jeff, so I have to go. I'll call you in the morning. Have a good night. I love you."

* * *

The four years ensuing my grandpa's death were demanding emotionally and mentally. When you're making 5 phone calls a day to remind someone to take medication, it's very easy to fall into the trap of dismissing it as another task to cross off the list. But this was my grandma and I didn't know how much longer she was going to be alive. I needed to spend as much quality time with her as I could, even if it was only over the phone. Jeff reminded me to stop and listen. To appreciate the texture in her voice, the tickle in her laugh, and the compassion in her advice; even in her frame of mind she offered love and support when I would complain about the state of my career—or lack thereof.

I was making fewer trips to Colorado. I was busy and I used that as an excuse, but in reality each trip was becoming more and more excruciating. The last Christmas I spent with her was the most unpleasant. This once magnificent woman with whom I would bake Christmas cookies, trade political dialogue, explore museums, dance around the living room, and sing carols with as a child, couldn't even swallow a glass of eggnog or sit still in a reclining chair while we unwrapped her presents.

I could see her mind working to engage in a conversation or react to a funny moment, and misfire. She was in agony. Her tremors were taking over and becoming much more intense. Oftentimes she would be thrown from the chair that she was sitting in and be stuck gnarled on the floor at the mercy of someone who would help her back to safety. She was taking the maximum dosage of medicine and it was no longer working. All we could do from that point on was watch her deteriorate.

The week before my 35th birthday, and my gram's 77th, I returned home for a visit. From our daily conversations I could tell that my grandma's health was declining. Nearly a year had passed since the last time I had visited her, and even then, it was emotionally draining and brutal to endure. Simple tasks like buttoning up a jacket or preparing a cup of tea could turn into a thirty-minute event. I avoided going home to face the truth at the expense of my grandma's feelings. I knew that a visit from me would help lift her spirits and provide a break for the rest of my family.

I arrived at my grandma's house with the best attitude I could invoke given the prospects. She opened the door to greet me and I gasped. Her smile was as jubilant as ever, but her frame was a blueprint of who she used to be; her once porcelain skin now shriveled and grey.

This was the same woman who, not that long before, would stand beside me in her kitchen and demonstrate her relevé and plié in perfect form as I would call upon the terminology she had learned in her childhood ballet lessons with Tony Genaro. I wondered if it was even safe to hug her. Before I had time to finish the question in my head, she released her clutch on the door handle—which was supporting her 78 pound frame—and hugged me tightly. She smelled exactly as she had my entire life—like a freshly cut rose.

I was ashamed of myself for waiting so long to visit. I was prepared to spend the next week indulging her to compensate for my delinquencies.

Immediately after I arrived in Colorado I concluded that things were far from satisfactory, and from what I could gather, the downturn had been significant over the past four months.

Why hadn't my dad called me sooner? We had an agreement. He swore he would be honest with me when the time came for me to escape the façade of sunlight and stardom that Hollywood pushes on dreamers. That evening dad and I discussed the situation over a long, sobering dinner.

The facts were: grandma had been gambling the ample allowance my dad provided her every week for lottery scratchers (compulsive gambling was *one* of the side effects of one of her Parkinson's drugs); after preparing her tea one morning, she had mistakenly left the burner on all day and a dishrag caught fire, thankfully a lifelong neighbor was there to save the day; and the worst was when she decided to walk two miles across town to the grocery store and on her way to Super Foods she forgot where she was headed. A police officer found my grandma wandering down the middle of Main Street. The officer was a friend of my sister, one of the benefits of living in a very small town, and he let my dad off without calling social services. He warned my dad that it was time to consider alternative living options; unfortunately my grandma refused to leave the house that she and my grandpa shared for fifty years.

My dad was in over his head. Even with the support from friends and my dad's wife, who took turns keeping a watchful eye on her while my dad was at work, my grandma's condition was becoming unmanageable without professional care.

Grandma and I spent the following morning catching up. She prepared herself a piece of toast with jelly and hot tea and glanced at the Denver Post. So far everything seemed normal, although she did mention several times that she wanted to stop by the Quick Stop to return her winning lottery tickets and buy more.

After her morning bath she got dressed and she was ready to "put on her face." A ritual that I'd enjoyed watching since I was a child; I sat next to her vanity as she applied her make-up. Only this time, she added her concealer after her foundation.

Finishing up her out-of-order make-up process, we discussed our plans for the rest of the day. She promptly reminded me that she needed to stop for more lottery scratchers.

It took us twenty minutes to get out of the house. Ten minutes to find her keys, which were hiding in the refrigerator, and ten minutes to collect all of the lottery tickets she had stashed around the house. On our way to lunch we stopped at Quick Stop to cash in.

We sat in the parked car outside the gas station calculating how much money my grandma had to collect. By my observation she hadn't won anything, but according to her knowledge of scratchers, she said she won $75. We disagreed and she was becoming flustered so I suggested that we take them to the counter; reminding her that the attendant inside would scan each ticket to verify if there were any winning tickets.

One by one the kid behind the counter scanned the tickets and handed them back. Just as I had suspected, there were no winners. My grandma's agitation developed into a panic and confusion. She pulled out $20 from her purse, dropping several bills of varying denominations onto the floor, handed the clerk the money and asked for more scratchers.

I picked up her scattered money that was littering the floor and handed it back to her. I informed her that she needed to be more careful and pointed her to a zippered pocket in her handbag that she could safely store loose currency in. She asked me not to baby her—which I thought was a fair request—and we proceeded to the car.

Inside the car she accused the clerk of lying and stealing her money. I swore that he was not cheating her and proposed that she start playing her new tickets.

As we approached our next destination, another small town ten minutes north of gram's house, she had completely finished "playing" each of the twenty cards. Clearly, the "Parkinson's shake" had some fringe benefits.

We were already running late to meet my mom at the restaurant when she asked me to stop at another Quick Stop. Evidently, my grandma was a missing character in the *Ocean's 11* movie franchise; the seventy-seven-year old granny with a gambling problem who's ready and willing to be a part of the con.

"Gram, we just stopped at the gas station and bought $20 worth of lottery tickets and we're late meeting my mom—I'll take you again tomorrow."

"It's on the way, I'll just run in and run out!"

I chuckled out loud. Had my grandma suddenly turned into an Olympic sprinter? "No gram, I don't think you'll be that quick. And you've already spent $20 on tickets today."

"Matt, don't be like that. Just stop for gram, please?"

I was irked and my patience was running low. I'd been in town two days and still hadn't seen my mom.

"Gram, drop it, please. We just stopped for you. I'm hungry and I want to see my mom."

She sat in silent protest. Refusing to answer the questions I posed in order to change the topic and refresh the mood.

We found my mom already indulging in chips and salsa. Grandma had tattled on me before we even sat down. "Matt wouldn't stop for *my* scratchers."

My mom, grandma's ex-daughter-in-law, was sympathetic. She hugged gram and reprimanded me for show.

I was so hungry I barked at my mom. I explained what had just transpired prior to meeting up with her, and still she felt unsatisfied.

"Matthew, if it makes her happy, why wouldn't you stop?"

Mom's point was valid, but I reacted defensively and spent the rest of our lunch—and the entire car trip home—in a foul mood.

In hindsight, I'm heartsick that I didn't just enjoy the time that I had with my grandma, regardless of what she wanted to do or how she was behaving. I was so vanquished with the state of my grandma's mental and physical downturn that I was trying to control the circumstances and force my grandma to be the woman she was before the Parkinson's diagnosis.

The battle with my grandma raged on once we got back to her house when my grandma accused my dad of withholding her money.

My dad, an only child, was now the executor of her estate and she didn't understand the seriousness of her implications. He was giving her a weekly allowance and managing her household bills. I questioned what my dad might have to gain; he had a house of his own and a wonderful job—he didn't need *her* money. I pointed out that she was probably spending more money on lottery tickets than she realized. My observation was not well received.

The same dazzling, rational, and scholarly woman who had helped me write my eighth grade commencement speech, advised me through my financial debacles in my early twenties, and counseled me on matters of faith and the heart, was gone. So was my patience.

What started out as a calm explanation rapidly escalated into a five-minute character assassination directed at her lack of logic. When I took a breath from my word annihilation this fragile, frightened soul stood there—still—like an exposed baby bunny during hunting season. Suddenly, she was herself again. She made direct eye contact with me and shared her anguish. All she said was, "Matt." In a tone that was both devastated and still compassionate. I hated myself.

In my lifetime, my grandma had been the only person who had never hurt me—ever. In the hour she needed me most, I responded with selfishness. The only way that I will ever escape the painful image of her reaction to my betrayal is if one day I face my own dementia. Even in that moment I realized my grandma was mentoring me; how to be kind, how to find compassion, how to listen, and how to forgive.

On the last day of my visit she was having a very good day and I was able to gain a fresh perspective and achieve some sense of peace. I seized the moment.

Fighting back tears and snot, I thanked her for showering me with endless love, guidance, wisdom, and inspiration. I praised her for her limitless support that led me to every victory and nourished me through every failure. I celebrated what a brilliant mother and grandmother she was, and vowed that I would never forget her spirit.

I looked deep into her eyes and I could still see the same woman who introduced me to my first library book, taught me how to be comfortable in my own skin, and gave me the permission to follow my heart, even when it meant moving 3,000 miles away from home.

Her reply was simple and honest, "That's what grandmas were made for."

We embraced for a long time, and I asked her if she could still dance with me.

"Of course!" She grabbed me by my waist and held on. Her feet began to step touch and sway side to side. I was delighted. We danced; I cried.

Suddenly she stopped and released me. She looked down at her leg and started shaking it rapidly, simulating the movement that takes over her body when she's having a tremor. "See, it even helps me dance!" she chuckled, referring to her disease. I pulled her in tight and joined in her laughter.

That was the most brilliant thing about my gram, no matter what the circumstance might bring, she never let life get her down.

She held me and whispered in my ear, "You've got talent, Matthew, *they* just haven't discovered you yet!"

My grandma passed away a month later. That was the last time I saw her alive.

Is It Safe To Come Out?

At five years old I had my entire life mapped out. I knew that I would be on television—and then—then all my dreams would come true. In middle school I fantasized what my life would be like when I was rich and famous. In every adaptation of the story I saw myself standing on a red carpet with a stunning wife by my side, just like my Hollywood heroes; Tom Cruise and Nicole Kidman, John Travolta and Kelly Preston, or Hugh Jackman and what's her name? Okay, I can see where my vision was askew. My childhood was vexed with the yearning to be normal, or at the very least, be perceived as normal.

Before I came out, I endured countless sleepless nights staring at the ceiling above my bed, exhausting my mind and agonizing over how my life would play out. Lying on a foldout futon in our shoebox apartment next to a girl whom—against my better judgment—I'd just moved across the country to play house with. I conjured up renditions of my life in the closet: me with my trophy wife, our two children who received their mother's porcelain skin, my thick hair, our combined eyes and high-cheek bones, and my vibrant acting career. It was everything I'd ever planned; however I knew I'd never fully enjoy this *Leave It To Beaver* moment, because I was living a dreadful lie.

Alternate late night scenarios explored the evolution of a life out of the closet. A depiction of my life where I was in a joyful, insatiable relationship with a strong, handsome, talented man who possessed Brad Pitt's looks; George Clooney's style; Colin Farrell's sexual appetite;

Will Ferrell's sense of humor; and Bill Clinton's charismatic drive and intelligence. Together, we would cook, travel the world, read literature, and discuss politics. Our weekends would be stacked doing home improvements, spa dates, operas, and the theater. We would spend hours in art museums debating the importance of pop art. No matter how hard I tried, I could not see how this fairytale fraternity of two would reconcile with my Hollywood ambition.

Inevitably, the driving necessity to come out of the closet and into reality exposed itself in the form of a perfect male silhouette wearing Prada. After a childhood full of confusion and shame; my teenage years full of repression and shame; and my early twenties filled with exploration, shame, elation, more shame, and finally heartbreak—I'd finally found the man of my dreams! It was love at first sight and I gave myself the permission to fall for him instantly and indefinitely.

Two years into our relationship, Jeff and I agreed that we would move back to Los Angeles. Looking back, I realize what a huge undertaking moving across the country can be for anyone, let alone two strong-willed, twenty-something men with Type-A personalities who were fresh on the gay scene. After taking inventory of our life in New York we concluded that our relationship could survive the journey.

In Los Angeles we quickly settled into a routine which included working out at the gym, spending too much money on food and entertainment, fighting about money, and struggling to find our way as actors in a town saturated with twenty-year-olds eager to be the next big thing.

Respectively we both had a lot of growing up to do, and while we no doubt quibbled a great deal, we both acknowledge that we loved one another and agreed to "do the work."

I was certain that I had found my match—then and now—Jeff possesses a quality which silently and lovingly demands constant awareness, intelligence, and creativity. In turn, I passionately provoked a fearless, relentless energy that challenged his responsible character. We feed off each other and once we learned how to harness and distribute our winning combination the bickering stopped and the creativity exploded.

Six years into our lives together, Jeff and I were focused on our creative journey. We had discussed marriage many times in our relationship and we knew that one day we wanted to throw a lavish wedding in Maui with all of the bravado that you'd expect from two chorus-boys-turned-Hollywood-power-couple. Of course we'd both committed ourselves to one another and planned on growing old together; we just accepted that we had work to do before our *Super Skinny Fabulous Gay Wedding* came.

I'll openly admit that I had become blissfully delusional while living "out of the closet" in Los Angeles, and I had let my gay-guard down. Here I was finally living the life of my dreams in a world that appeared so much more accepting than it had been during my childhood. So, on November 4, 2008 my soul was decimated learning that California's Proposition 8 had passed, making it impossible (and illegal) for same-sex couples to get married. I was thirty and being bullied back into the closet by an entire group of misinformed or uncompassionate voters.

All of the rage, anxiety, and despair I felt throughout my adolescence had resurfaced, only now I was unflinching in my readiness to take action. Marching, preaching, social media posting, and creating work that would challenge people to see past a stereotype and confront the truth: people who fall in love with people of the same sex are people too.

From that day on, Jeff and I vowed that no matter where we were in life, if (when) the opportunity for same-sex couples to get married presented itself (again), we would act without hesitation and tie-the-knot pronto.

On June 26, 2013 the federal court decision, which ruled Prop 8 unconstitutional, went into effect. Three days later my grandma passed away. It was the most bittersweet time in my life. I was conflicted with simultaneous feelings of elation and anguish, and everything in between.

I was traveling extensively at the time, so Jeff and I spent the majority of our "quality time" on the phone. Sitting in airports or random Hyatt Places across the United States we exchanged our life events, discussed our business matters, and attempted *sexy* time, in the form of text messaging tastefully, *artistic* pictures of our leg or the side of our neck and shoulder, because neither one of us is a Millennial willing to "accidentally" expose our penis to the void we call the internet.

In between snapping selfies and balling my brains out, Jeff and I both mentioned marriage. In unison we agreed that between burying my grandma in Colorado and choreographing a gig in Branson, MO, I would fly back to Los Angeles for two days and we would sashay down to Beverly Hills City Hall.

Was it ideal that I would so quickly, but still mindfully, be saying my final goodbyes to the woman who ultimately shaped my entire life and shared her unending love and support, before swiftly rushing off to Los Angeles to marry the man whom I would enter the most important contract of endless love, support, laughter, and creativity with? NO. But it happened that way all the same.

After losing my grandpa I recognized how quickly life can change and it inspired a surge of creativity, fearlessness, and determination; I had nothing to lose. When I lost my grandma, I thought—now what? She was my constant source of motivation and suddenly she was gone. I had two choices: I could let my spirit die with her or I could celebrate the legacy that she left me and monopolize every single day.

We arrived early in Beverly Hills on Friday July 12, 2013. We were the third couple in line waiting to pick up our wedding licenses. In the twenty minutes that we stood waiting for the courthouse doors to open, the line expanded into something you might expect when Barbra Streisand announces her "final" concert. Jeff called ahead, so we knew that we would be able to secure the license in one day, but because of the overwhelming number of LGBTQ couples eager to enter into a blissful life of monogamy, there was a two week wait. In short, we would not be able to get married at the courthouse.

Always resourceful, we reached out to one of our closest friends, who was an ordained minister and stand-up comedian. Amy had already married off two other couples whom we were close with and we knew that she would bring our special day to life in that unique way that only a Southern Belle turned hilariously talented liberal-environmentalist-stand-up-comedian who also marries friends could.

We decided that with the exception of our parents and a handful of our friends, we wouldn't tell anyone that we were getting married. We still wanted to have a lavish wedding celebration down the road, so we would keep this a simple ceremony celebrating our love and guaranteeing the ability to care for one another in the event that, God forbid, either of us ended up in a hospital.*

---

*   Let's not forget that a plethora of emergency rooms denied same-sex couples

Word of our secret ceremony was passed faster than a hallucinogen at Coachella and so we decided that we would post one abstract picture of the rings we had just purchased at Tiffany & Co. (naturally) with a vague caption. Anyone who reached out to us privately with questions would be privy to the details.

It turns out that we actually had a large group of friends who cared about us enough to dig deeper for answers and so by go time, we knew to expect about 40 invited guests.

I use the word *invited* because we decided to capitalize on the free Jazz Night that the Los Angeles County Museum of Art presents every Friday evening throughout the summer. Unbeknownst to the entire LACMA staff at precisely 3:30 p.m. on Friday July 12, 2013, Jeff and I arrived with our friend Ari, who purchased a last minute airline ticket from New York City to join us, and laid our claim on a valuable grassy section of the exquisitely maintained courtyard.

With matching blankets, vinyl picnic tablecloths that we purchased from the Ninety-Nine Cents store (yes, gays can be resourceful—AKA—cheap), color-coordinated helium balloons, and periwinkle potted Hydrangeas; we locked off the northwest corner of the grounds. Jeff chose the spot next to a towering red sculpture and just behind the new wing of the museum ensuring a superb spot within earshot of the jazz band, a sweeping view of the palm tree lined streets, a panoramic shot of the Hollywood Hills, and ample shade when the sun is at its peak.

Unsuspecting LACMA patrons stormed the grounds staking claim around our soon-to-be wedding venue. Our guests started arriving with cheer, gifts, and bottles of champagne. One of the most unpredictable moments was when our straight friend, Lee, presented us with two "Groom" cake toppers—which was brilliant—because, while Jeff made a delectable homemade spiced cake with the most magnificent cream cheese frosting, we hadn't the time to amass the traditional décor. Our thoughtful friend, Lee and his wife, Bevin, who also came in tow with an ice chest full of fancy bubbly, saved our bad gay moment!

the right to spend the final moments of their spouse's life by their side, because while they might have spent thirty years of their lives together and in many instances had children and homes together, they were not legally recognized by our government as family members; and in many cases left penniless despite wills and wishes.

An hour into the jazz, after we greeted our guests and shared the rationale behind our "zany" last minute nuptials, we started the ceremony. Did I mention that our minister, Amy, also had a stand-up set later that evening? We had to get the ball-and-chain rolling.

We found our moment when the jazz musicians took a fifteen-minute intermission. Amy stood up and faced our friends. My heart was racing and I was full of joy. I hadn't expected to feel so emotional, but here I was standing next to Jeff with a group of our friends and suddenly I watched a highlight reel of my life with Jeff flash across the cloudless deep blue sky above.

Amy started the scene with a pun, because Jeff loves a pun, and Amy aims to please. She continued to share a heartfelt story that was funny and poignant, which she had composed in a day.

The moment came to say, "I do", and I stood there with a substantial amount of tears in my eyes. I took deep breaths and focused on the ecstasy radiating off Jeff. Our puppies Lily the Shih tzu and Ginger the Yorkie, escorted by our friends Maggie and Bevin, were the ring bearers. I took the ring and stared into Jeff's eyes. The world went silent, my body began to experience a warm euphoric tingling and I felt like I was floating; I am not a romantic and yet there I was gushing with unexplainable gratitude.

When Amy, whose vocal projection had gradually increased during her delivery making good on her USC theater degree, announced us as husband and husband, an explosion of cheers and deafening applause enveloped us. I snapped back from my out-of-body experience and slowly took inventory of the scene. In every direction men, women, and children who had come to enjoy an evening of music and merriment had decidedly become extended guests at our wedding. Like every Italian wedding, strangers we'd never met came to offer their congratulations, advice, and love.

Men charged over to shake our hands and wish us luck. Women approached us with tears and open arms ready for hugs. Children invited themselves to our cake and balloons.

Standing next to his fussy wife, one man confessed, "I wish she would have planned a wedding like this." A lesbian couple thanked us for the powerful statement, demonstrating how natural it is for same-sex couples to be married. An older couple stopped by to share their secret for 50 years of bliss together. The wife said, "We never fight." Her husband confessed, "We fight all the time." The generous emotional support continued throughout the evening. Random people airdropped videos and photos that they took for us. Children—high on the sugar from the cake they demolished—danced around cheerfully while music and laugher vibrated across the plaza.

After years of deflecting devastating schoolyard slurs, supermarket slanders, self-inflicted hate, Hollywood hesitations, and outright intolerance; despite my growth, self-acceptance, and declarations of Pride, as the sunset cast a splendid golden hue on the man who was offering me a lifetime of unconditional love, support, creativity, and enduring laughter; there before God, The Universe, many of our closest friends, and several hundred Los Angelinos who were out for a festive evening of jazz and unwittingly participated in the only Flash-wedding the Los Angeles County Museum of Art has ever officially, unofficially hosted, I finally had the answer to my most insistent question: "Is it safe to come out?" The answer for me was simply and unambiguously, yes.

CPSIA information can be obtained
at www.ICGtesting.com
Printed in the USA
BVHW052238020919
557385BV00007B/112/P

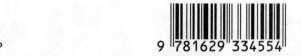